the Martini Diet

the Martini Diet

The Self~Indulgent Way to a Thinner, More Fabulous You!

JENNIFER "GIN" SANDER

Author of *Wear More Cashmere: 151 Luxurious Ways to Pamper Your Inner Princess*
foreword by Martin G. Neft, M. D.

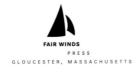

FAIR WINDS
PRESS
GLOUCESTER, MASSACHUSETTS

First published in the USA in 2004 by
Fair Winds Press
33 Commercial Street
Gloucester, MA 01930

08 07 06   2 3 4 5

ISBN-13: 978-1-59233-188-8
ISBN-10: 1-59233-188-2

Library of Congress Cataloging-in-Publication Data available

Cover and interior book design by
Laura McFadden Design, Inc.
laura.mcfadden@rcn.com

Cover and interior illustrations by
Carlos Marerro
www.marrero.net

Printed and bound in China

*The information in this book is for educational purposes only. It is not
intended to replace the advice of a physician or medical practitioner.
Please see your health care provider before beginning any new health program.*

*"If you obey all the rules,
you miss all the fun."*

—KATHARINE HEPBURN

In which The Martini Diet Indulgent Philosophy is introduced to you. The Martini Diet is about indulgence balanced with restraint. You are encouraged to become a complete food snob, rising above the dross that surrounds you, saving yourself to indulge in only the best.

Once you become a food snob, you will find that the higher your nose is in the air, the smaller your behind. Snacking must go, as it simply isn't elegant. Portion control will become critical—if it doesn't fit in a martini glass, you've served up too much food.

If you plan to indulge regularly and still be slim, you must also plan to move. But not everyone is cut out for Pilates and Bikram Yoga. There are other, more indulgent ways to exercise. Ice skating, horseback riding, and fencing are other elegant ways to get in shape.

Learn why you really should drink wine and liquor (scientific reasons!) and a few equally scientific reasons why chocolate doesn't have to be eliminated from the Martini Diet.

Contents

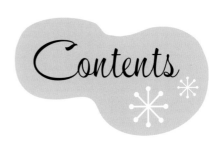

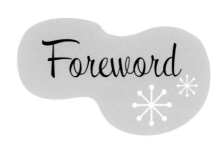

Foreword

IS THERE ANYTHING IN THE HEALTH FIELD MORE FRUSTRATING than the battle to lose weight? As a family physician, I regularly hear desperate pleas from patients for help in their battle against their weight. I will be asked about medications. Maybe you have a pill that will help me get started? How about the latest diet that helped their neighbor lose 25 pounds in a month? And I know that all too often, the promise of this month's fix will prove to be illusory. Those pills all have serious downsides, and only work when you are taking them. Most diets work at first but it turns out to be nearly impossible to keep for sustained periods. Beating ourselves up and torturing ourselves just doesn't seem to work.

Gin's Martini Diet offers a refreshing, and promising approach. She tells us to find things we enjoy, and indulge, but in moderation. It's an approach that certainly makes psychological as well as physiological sense, and it's worked for her. Gin is reminding us of one principle of diet management that we know is essential—you must adopt a lifestyle change that you can sustain. And you only will be able to sustain it if it brings you pleasure. For those of you tired of torturing yourselves with potent medications or rigid self-denial, consider this approach. Indulge yourself. And keep it up. It may just work!

— MARTIN NEFT, M.D.

Introduction

Y

When the day came for me to turn in the manuscript for the lovely little book *Wear More Cashmere: 151 Luxurious Ways to Pamper Your Inner Princess*, Paula, my editor, flipped through the pages, read a few entries, and sighed out loud. "It's lovely. I look forward to living this way. You know what's on my mind nowadays, though? My inner princess has such a big butt. Isn't there a way for me to indulge and pamper myself and somehow end up wearing cashmere in a slightly smaller size?"

"Without question," I said, delighted to be asked. I'd long dreamed of the day when someone, somewhere, would ask me for my diet and beauty secrets. In high school, I had a ready answer—guacamole. Of course my glowing skin, shiny hair, and classic cheerleader figure came from California-grown avocados!

Time passed, as did my youthful ability to eat absolutely anything and still shop in the junior department. Older and wiser now, I say the answer is gin.

Gin, you ask? Yes, gin, in the form of a glistening martini. A martini symbolizes all that I seek in life—the simple, the elegant, the refined. And, I confess, the slightly sinful. A dry gin martini presented in a crystal glass beaded with icy little drops of water. So very tall, so very thin; two things I've long aspired to. The height is easy enough to acquire: I just slip into my 3½-inch Jimmy Choo mules and I'm as tall as a supermodel. The thinness thing, well, that is *much* harder to acquire.

There came a day when I looked in the mirror at my forty-year-old self and thought—this is not *at all* what I had in mind. Compounding the feelings of annoyance that came from viewing myself in a full-length mirror was the news I'd just received from my gym. It seemed my longtime personal trainer, Mario, had been fired. For making passes at his female clients. Hmmm. What did it mean, that in two years, Mario had never made a pass at *me*? I vowed then and there to permanently change my eating habits in order to permanently change my appearance.

While developing the philosophy and attitude my editor Paula eventually christened "the Martini Diet," my body truly has changed. By modifying the way I think and behave, I've finally dropped those dumpy ten pounds. In these pages, you'll find my food philosophy and ideas to help you get closer to the way you want *your* body to look for life. Isn't it time you escaped the cycle of self-loathing, guilt, and dieting failures that seem to dog us all, and indulge in delicious, real food, while changing the way your body looks? Of course it is.

And yes, in this little book you will find weight loss for the self-indulgent. Let's get this straight right from the beginning—I'm not a diet doctor. I'm not a nutritionist. I'm a nonscientist, to put it kindly. What I am is a self-indulgent and naturally curvy woman who would prefer to sit idly in a beachside lounge chair while cabana boys bring me cool drinks. Instead I work hard every day to stay loose inside of a pair of size six Calvin Klein jeans (I've long suspected they were mismarked, but why check the tag on a gift horse?), while still hoping to squeeze my share of pleasure out of every day.

I'm sensing the need to define my terms here. You may well wonder just what this book means by the tantalizing subtitle, "The Self-Indulgent Way to a Thinner More Fabulous You!" Indulgence is not a synonym for gluttony—far from it. It is simply the absence of fear when it comes to allowing yourself a pleasure, combined with the courage to declare that, henceforth, you will allow only the very best of everything into your life. Be warned that I will soon recommend taking these pleasures in modest helpings, though. Perhaps we can describe it as "grace under pleasure."

In *Wear More Cashmere*, I extolled the pleasures of taking charge of your own happiness and creating the kind of life you want for yourself. Do you long for a life of small luxuries and delicious indulgence? Rather than sitting idly by and waiting for someone else to give them permission, women need to decide that they deserve to be pampered, to indulge themselves with the very best.

You deserve to rise above the suburban sameness that surrounds us in modern life and hold out for something different and unique. It won't happen unless you make the decision, unless you make it happen on your own. That same "cashmere attitude" should extend to your weight and your body. You deserve to eat the food you want, rather than constantly denying yourself the best life has to offer. So why sit there waiting?

You won't find me waiting. You'll find me at my favorite table at Morton's of Chicago, martini glass firmly in hand, happily contemplating the menu and trying to decide between the prime rib or the rib eye.

Don't imagine the Martini Diet only involves indulging in wonderful food and doesn't involve working up a sweat on a regular basis. It does indeed. Exercise is a major element in the Martini lifestyle. Recognizing, however, that not every woman longs to sweat in a Bikram studio or stretch on a Pilates machine (and you can include me in that group), I've devoted a whole chapter to more indulgent types of exercise.

Here's a little something to consider, darlings: Americans spend more than thirty-three billion dollars a year on weight-loss products and services. Imagine how many more cashmere sweaters, vintage fur coats, massages and other pampering delights we could all indulge in if we just adopted my eating and lifestyle advice and dispensed with this nonsense once and for all. No more exercise machines, no more expensive food plans. Life is full to the brim of possibility and delicious opportunity. I think you should be getting a big taste of both, don't you?

Let's begin. Pour yourself a tall and thin martini now, settle your indulgent self in a comfortable chair, and read on to adopt a new, more luxurious attitude toward weight loss and lifetime weight maintenance.

Yours with a lemon twist,

JENNIFER "GIN" SANDER

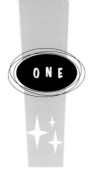

ONE

Shaken, Not Stirred
The indulgent philosophy

Wouldn't life be grand if we could eat absolutely anything we wanted, spend our leisure-filled days lying on cool satin sheets reading novels and our nights being romanced by tuxedo-clad investment bankers? Indeed, that life would be grand, but I'm afraid this is only a dream. Real life can include some of these things in smallish doses, such as the silky sheets and perhaps at least one man in a tuxedo (alas, most likely rented). As for eating absolutely anything we want, well, in smallish doses that can be true, too.

The basic idea behind the Martini Diet is *indulgence* balanced with *restraint*. Where does that idea come from, you ask? From the empty-glass side of a thousand martinis, my dears. Because when drinking gin, you must be restrained indeed. Just one of those tall, thin, elegantly clear glasses of gin decorated with just a twist of tart lemon is the perfect amount. If you had two martinis you might do something silly. If you had three martinis, you might well do something you'd regret and end up splashed all over the newspapers for your neighbors to giggle over in the morning. Dorothy Parker, a tart-tongued member of the famed Round Table at the Algonquin Hotel in New York during the witty 1930s, summed up the problem this way:

> *I like to have a martini,*
> *Two at the very most.*
> *Three I'm under the table,*
> *Four I'm under the host.*

Sounds like a reasonable attitude we should extend into other areas of life, doesn't it? One of something is delightful, two should be a rare treat, and beyond that small number, danger lies. In fact, if we just switch Parker's martinis to, say, ice cream, the same warning still holds true:

> *I like to eat Ben & Jerry's,*
> *Just one scoop to tickle my lips.*
> *Two scoops will make me feel sluggish,*
> *Three and it stays on my hips.*

Clearly I'm not in the same league with the late Mrs. Parker, but you see the wisdom of this, don't you?

The title of this book is *The Martini Diet: The Self-Indulgent Way to a Thinner, More Fabulous You!*. I'm guessing you picked it up because the words *self-indulgent* struck you as an all too accurate description of yourself. Why not add to that description and include a few more selves in that image—let's add *self-possessed* and *self-confident*. You and I indulge because we are confident enough to believe that we are entitled to what life has to offer; we aren't shy about stepping up and smiling and accepting what has been offered. In this cruel, cruel world, we need all the self-possession and self-confidence we can muster up!

Our Bodies, Ourselves

Before I begin to win you over to the Martini Diet philosophy, let me first climb daintily up on my soapbox and speak to you about women's bodies. There are so very many wonderful things about being a woman: We can do things like wear expensive lace underwear, read trashy romance novels, highlight our hair, and, best of all, prance around in vaguely trampy sandals in the summertime. Not everything about being a woman is so easy, though. Everywhere we turn—every magazine, newspaper, movie, or television show—someone is trying hard to undermine how we feel about our bodies.

The Martini Diet isn't just about how you eat, it is also about how *you* feel about *your* body. And as you will learn in the coming chapters, it is also about turning up your nose at much of the junkier aspects of life, from fast food to fast eating. I want you to start lifting your nose in the air now by rising above the media messages about what a perfect body looks like.

Inasmuch as I cling to the mental image of a martini glass as my bodily *ne plus ultra*, I am never going to be called skinny. After four decades in this body, I'm okay with that.

Now the soapbox speech begins: I'm standing up here today to tell you that you need to become immune to Madison Avenue's image of how women should look, of how *you* should look. As you embrace the Martini Diet philosophy, you will also need to develop the ability to ignore most food advertising, too. The combination of image after image of tiny little women in tiny little clothes and image after image of cheesecake, cheeseburgers, and cheese puffs will drive you mad.

I'll let you in on an industry secret—here is what lies behind those beautifully photographed and stylized images that surround us: There are armies of well-paid advertising execs who stay up late at night thinking of ways to get you to buy more of their product (often only by first making you feel that, sigh, your life is empty without it). The galling twist when it comes to our bodies and food is this—there are a bunch of smart and creative folks whose job is to make you feel like your life is lacking because you don't own a pair of bright blue leather jeans, and until you walk into a department store and buy a pair, you'll feel hopelessly empty. There is an equally smart and talented bunch who devote themselves to creating compelling advertising to make you feel that once you sink your teeth into a stuffed-crust pizza, your life will be forever fulfilled.

Even a nonscientist like me can do the math on this one—you can't eat the pizza and still fit into the leather jeans in that teeny tiny size. So you are doomed, doomed, doomed. If you absorb the message from one advertiser you can't succumb to the other. Both messages together conspire to leave you restless and dissatisfied with what you already have, whether it is a pair of ordinary jeans you just bought last week or a healthy fresh salad that suddenly doesn't look nearly as enticing now that you've got stuffed-crust pizza on your mind.

What to do? Vow that henceforth (vowing anything and using the word "henceforth" makes it stick better) you will not allow *any* advertisers to make you feel inadequate. You will not allow any advertising to convince *you* that your life is empty without their product. Your life is full. The next time you see a 100-pound girl model a pair of teeny jeans, the next time you see an ad in a magazine for eye cream that features a sixteen year old, the next time you see an ad for a glistening piece of frozen cheesecake, you will nod sagely and think—ha! Did a marketing executive really think I was dumb enough to fall for that? *Puhleeze*.

Jennifer Lopez's Bottom

There does seem to be a glimmer of change on the media horizon. All the press attention given to actress/singer Jennifer Lopez's behind is a good sign, even though it still looks pretty smallish to me. Models whose bodies are size ten, twelve, and fourteen, instead of zero or two, are featured in the occasional advertising campaign. But that still leaves the eights and tens among us feeling like odd girls out. I'm here to say that if you are an eight or a ten I encourage you to adopt the Martini Diet lifestyle for your long-term health, but not because you've been made to believe your body is hopelessly huge. It isn't. You are perfectly (and I do mean perfectly) normal.

Radical as I am sounding here, I am not at all pro-fat. I won't pretend that in our world really big women are for the most part either happy or healthy. My own best friend of many years, Laura, was a big, big girl, and it made my heart ache to see the looks she got from strangers. Sideways glances, shaking heads, and sneers from people who were making judgments about her based solely on her size. Thinness is prized in our world, and I won't pretend otherwise. If you follow the Martini Diet, I firmly believe that you will be thinner and healthier as a result. But please, please don't begin your diet because you want to be a size two.

To prepare to play the chunky lead in the Bridget Jones movies, tiny Renée Zellweger packed on a well-publicized twenty pounds or so. And at that monstrous weight she *still* weighs fifteen pounds less than I do! So it is a losing battle; you will never be satisfied or happy with your body if that is who you are trying to emulate. Don't make yourself crazy by choosing the wrong role model. Begin now to unhook that part of your brain that absorbs and internalizes those images. By the end of this book, you will not be moved by the sight of the Golden Arches; neither will you feel inadequate when your gaze falls upon the carefully airbrushed and crafted image of a perfect model in a magazine spread. Living the Martini Diet lifestyle is a sophisticate's choice, and sophisticated women like you and me make extremely sophisticated choices about our food and drink, and we are equally sophisticated about media manipulation. *Oui?*

The Real American Idol

I am much influenced by the great style icons of the past, women such as longtime *Vogue* editor Diana Vreeland and chic Parisian designer Coco Chanel. Much as I idolize and adore these two, and also women such as Jackie Onassis and Wallis Windsor, they are just too skinny for my taste. Flip through the biographies of some of these women and it seems they didn't eat at all. Mostly they smoked and drank cups of bouillon for lunch and dinner. Cigarettes and clear beef broth? Not at all my cup of tea. Fond as I am of the occasional cigar, tobacco has never appealed to me as a method of weight control. In book after book, I searched for evocative and inspiring accounts of lavish late-night banquets in grand candlelit dining rooms, but it seemed the focus was more often on what hung in their closets than what was prepared in their kitchens. These dazzling women are still my idols when it comes to decorating a house with puffy chintz pillows or choosing an outfit to wear to the opera, but when trying to develop a lifetime eating plan, I wasn't inspired to imitate their habits.

The Martini Lifestyle

Wallis, the Duchess of Windsor, was the very woman who coined the familiar phrase "*You can never be too rich or too thin.*" Sorry Wallis, dear, you *can* be too thin.

So there I was, dumpy at forty, unhappy with the way my jeans fit, yet equally unhappy contemplating a life in which I had to give up so much of what I loved in order to be thin. Surely there was some other role model out there with a sensible yet sensuous attitude toward a dinner plate?

And then suddenly, I found her. The very role model I was seeking. She had been a part of my life since childhood. How had I overlooked her in my search for guidance? An accomplished woman with a long string of successes, one who was able to incorporate a love of good food into a healthy lifestyle and a normal weight. Who was this goddess? None other than the queen of American food herself, the inimitable Julia Child.

Scrambling up on my soapbox once again (so difficult to do in a ladylike manner), I urge you all to abandon your foolish admiration of the superthin Cindy Crawfords and Kate Mosses of the modeling world. Instead, let's all sit adoringly at the feet of Julia Child, who rose to prominence in her early fifties as public television's French chef. Was it because she was thin and beautiful and looked fabulous in front of a camera? No, it was because she was a smart and funny woman with a terrific and level-headed attitude toward food. Toward making food, and just as important, toward *eating* food. You might well know of Julia Child from television and her best-selling cookbooks. Allow me to fill you in on her unique eating philosophy.

Described by *Gourmet* magazine as an unashamed evangelist for butter and cream, Julia is opposed to any product or recipe positioned as "no-fat," which she describes as "a process, not a food." In her many decades on public television, Julia taught America how to enjoy food. You'd think we already knew how to do that, wouldn't you?

Although Julia McWilliams Child was born and raised in Pasadena, California, her food training and experience came from years of living in Paris with her husband, Paul. A stint at the famed cooking school *Cordon Bleu* led her to spend ten years developing the cookbook *Mastering the Art of French Cooking* along with two friends.

When asked by the hoards of interviewers who descended upon the occasion of her ninetieth birthday in the summer of 2002 just why she believed she'd led a long and healthy life, Julia revealed her secret, "red meat and gin." Most any type of gin will do, she thinks, but she prefers Gordon's as her own top pick. Red meat and gin as the secret to long life? My heart pounded as I read these promising words. Does it get any better than that? It isn't just red meat and gin that does the trick, of course; it's also eating in moderation. Julia told *Esquire* magazine that moderation, small helpings, and sampling a little bit of everything are the secrets to good health and happiness. Not a snacker, she isn't totally impervious to the charms of junk food. "I don't eat between meals. I don't snack. Well, I do eat those little fish crackers. They're fattening, but irresistible."

The Science of Self-Indulgence

Red meat was painted as a dangerous item for much of the previous decades, but science has redeemed it. Not only is it a terrific source of protein, zinc, and iron, red meat is also the best source of certain B vitamins. Julia Child knows whereof she speaks.

Let's sum up Julia's philosophy this way—eat wonderful food, take modest portions, and skip the snacking between meals. Do those sound like simple and elegant food rules you can live by? They sounded pretty attractive to me. How much of Julia's attitude toward food and eating was influenced by her years in France? No doubt a good deal of it, as her rules mirror the way most of those Parisian women we envy for their style and poise eat every day. In the next chapter, you will learn more about the eating habits of the French and how we can put them to work in our own American lives.

A final thought on what else made Julia Child succeed on television in the sixties. Russell Morash was her producer for many decades, and he shares this thought: "She was a gifted scholar, she knew her stuff, and she was confident at a time when women generally weren't." Even though I've already gently nudged you once on this topic I will do it again—it will take confidence to decide that you will begin to eat in a way your friends and family might not understand. Confidence is another delicious ingredient Julia would have us use often.

The Science of Self-Indulgence

Alors, the "French Paradox" is mind boggling. How can those folks eat croissants, cheeses, and sausages, drink glass after glass of wine and still be so chic and slim? Despite their rich cuisine, the French are much, much slimmer than the citizens of our beloved nation: 30 percent of Americans are obese, but only 8 percent of the French fall into that category. Anyone want to join me and buy a one-way ticket to Paris?

Get Up Off of That Thing

I've already warned you that indulgence is not gluttony, that on the Martini Diet you will not be diving face first into a tub of Häagen-Dazs every morning. If indulgence is not gluttony, neither is it indolence. By adopting the Martini Diet, you will be increasing the activity in your life, not increasing the amount of time you spend lying about reading fashion magazines. Far from it. If you want to maintain a slim and healthy body weight, you've got to get up and move.

Have you ever read one of those maddening articles about a supermodel or a famous actress who shrugged off the suggestion that she works at her beauty? Any professional in the entertainment business who says the words "I eat whatever I want" is stretching the truth. The brilliant and beautiful actress and producer, Salma Hayak, says, "I eat pork, and I love my red wine," but she also says she doesn't exercise. Darn it all, Salma, much as I want to believe you, I'm suspicious.

It takes hours of work in the gym day in and day out to appear in a magazine or on the red carpet at the Oscars. And just like the maddening messages we all receive from advertisements for food, clothing, and cosmetics, the idea that any of us can be slim and in shape without exercise has sent more than one frustrated dieter back to the fridge. We all want to appear as though our lives are effortless. How crass to be seen actually *working* at something. And to be seen working at something as shallow as toning your body would seem even more crass to most people. To embrace the Martini Diet, you *will* have to work at it. It isn't as unpleasant as I make it sound, of course.

The Science of Self-Indulgence

Exercise not only keeps your behind from jiggling, but it also makes your food taste better. Really. According to the *European Journal of Clinical Nutrition*, women who exercise regularly are less likely to snack and munch between meals, and they take greater pleasure from what they do eat.

Put Your Nose in the Air

"Now don't be a snob, dear," your mother said over and over as you were growing up. Very good advice your mother was giving, but I want you to try to overcome that little voice in your head. Yes, what I want you to become is a *snob*. Not a snob toward other people, mind you, but truly a snob about what you eat. I encourage you to feel superior when confronted with a plate of gloppy macaroni salad, a bag of fast-food fries, or a birthday cake from a grocery store. Just think to yourself, "not quite good enough for me." Please don't say this out loud while passing through the banquet line at your best friend's carefully planned wedding reception, though; you and I both know that someone will end up crying. This is a quiet conversation you will hold with yourself, one that will become routine as you dispense with the edible dross that surrounds us. Try not to move your lips.

Becoming a food snob will make it remarkably easy to give up junk food. There is no question that it is not up to your very high standards, that it is far, far beneath you. In the next chapter, I'll delve more deeply into further convincing you just how appalling and unbecoming junk food really is.

Adopt this as your new credo—*Eat well, or not at all.* In fact, the more you know about food, the less you will eat of what is commonly available. You won't be tempted in the least by the waves of donuts and cookies that appear in your office every day. The average American consumes more than 150 pounds of sugar each year. Think about it, aren't those bags of sugar in the store five pounds each? So we each consume THIRTY of those bags per year? That is an appalling enough image to turn us all off cake and cookies forever. Simply cutting back on sugary foods will make you feel immensely superior to the person standing next to you in line at the grocery store with a cart full of muffins and Pop Tarts.

When I use the word "indulge," when I talk about indulging, I am not talking about indulging in one of those tacky Pop Tarts or an extra large bag of fries. I want you to save your moments of indulgence (and there will be many once you learn to live this way) for the best that life has to offer—creamy soups, fresh fruit pies, soufflés, and perfectly roasted chickens. And one stellar martini, of course. Here is a simple way to sum up this theory— *the higher your nose is in the air about what you eat, the smaller your butt will be.*

Eat the Best While Wearing the Best

Over the years, as I developed the Martini Diet and eliminated substandard food from my meals, I also began to upgrade my wardrobe. Who wants to eat incredible food and drink expensive gin while wearing ordinary clothes?

My theme of indulgence balanced with restraint extends to your wardrobe too, my dears. Remember that standard old diet trick of buying something lovely and expensive in a smaller size to guilt yourself into losing weight and fitting into it? While living the Martini lifestyle, our credo is—don't wait, dear, buy something extraordinary now. As you do lose weight you can simply have it tailored to fit your new body— someone has to keep the tailors of the world employed. There is just no reason to deny yourself the very best, because regardless of your current weight, you deserve it already. Who knew that this wicked-sounding diet book would also turn out to be a shopping manifesto!

I've also found that indulging in beautiful clothes keeps me from eating too much sometimes. Not only do I want to be able to fit easily into those snug Escada sailor pants, but I also don't really want the huge dry cleaning bill I'd be faced with if I spilled taco sauce on my consignment-shop Chanel jacket. The posher my outfit, the lower the chance that I will order something that will end up splashing me. No wonder Jackie and Wallis were so darn thin—they too were trying to avoid mussing up a couture outfit.

Living the Martini Life

Don't feel discouraged when I toss around big designer names such as Chanel and Escada. I can't afford them either, yet they are hanging in my closet. My secret is that they are used. Some other woman paid full price for these treasures, wore them a few times, and then sent them off to a designer resale or consignment shop where I picked them up for a fraction of their original cost. A Chanel suit costs upward of $3,000, but the red suit I'm wearing to lunch today cost $250. If your town doesn't have a designer resale store, go online and see what you can find on eBay.

Born Again Sophisticate

And lastly, a big part of the Martini Diet philosophy involves attaining not just the weight and size you've long sought, but also the life you've long sought. When I was a little girl, my fantasy life revolved around the idea that I would grow up to be a stylish single woman of the world who lived in a glamorous big city apartment and raced around in an antique Jaguar. Funny thing, I never daydreamed about the kind of life I actually ended up having—the married mother of two boys, living in the California suburbs, picking up an endless stream of dirty socks off the floor, and nagging everyone about homework.

In fact, as I considered my life late in the afternoon of my fortieth birthday, I was feeling pretty low. I've already told you how discouraged I was about my weight. My husband Peter, (the father of the boys with the dirty socks), and I were in a cute little boutique on the island of Hawaii (okay, so maybe it wasn't all bad) wandering among the tiny dresses on display. Nope, not my size, not my size, I thought, as I rifled through the racks. Then, just at the moment when I thought I couldn't feel worse about myself, the door to that cute little boutique in Hawaii opened and in walked... Bo Derek. That's right, the very moment I am feeling the lowest about my body, in walks the woman the whole world remembers as the perfect 10.

Well, you can imagine how well that went down with my ego. Dumpy suburban housewife Jennifer comes face to face with Bo Derek.

Hours later, I sat on the beach pouting about my fate. I didn't grow up to be that stylish and worldly single woman. Bo Derek did. And *Bo*? Even her name sounded more glamorous than mine did, I thought, sticking out my lip even further.

But wait! Her mother didn't name her Bo, her late husband did. Because it sounded dashing and glamorous. So if I didn't have the dashing and glamorous life I'd hoped for, maybe I could at least sound like I did. And there on the beach in Hawaii I decided that my name would be GIN. Not Jen, not Jenny, but Gin. While Jennifer is picking up those dirty socks, her alter ego Gin is off traveling the world in search of adventure and intrigue. And as you might have guessed, Gin is also the person who slimmed down for good.

Who did you want to be when you grew up? Perhaps you had a whole different idea of how your life would turn out. Most people do. So why not take this opportunity to rename yourself, to choose a name for the new you who is embarking on this new diet and will soon emerge with a new body and a new outlook on life. You can decide today to be someone else, even before you begin to adopt the Martini Diet lifestyle into your life.

Feel free to keep your new name a secret, or share it with a close friend or two. I only introduce myself as Gin on occasion. Gee, if I can call myself *Gin*, you can call yourself something equally outrageous. Try it and see whether it doesn't give you a new outlook on the life you have now.

My motto in life is **Wear More Cashmere!** Not only do I adore cashmere itself, of course, but to me it is also a wonderful metaphor for whatever it is that we seem to deny ourselves. "Oh no," you say, as someone offers you something wonderful in life, "I really shouldn't. . ." Yes, you really should. You really should create the life you want, and the body to go with it. Why pour yourself and your energies into others on an endless basis?

Have I got you charged up and ready to move on to the eating plan? I know you will be delighted to learn how easily you will be able to fold the Martini Diet into your everyday life.

Y

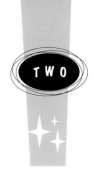

TWO

The Martini Diet
Indulgent Eating Plan

All the various diets you've tried over the years have yet to make a permanent dent in your denim size. Not to worry, Gin to the rescue! With Julia Child as our beloved food goddess and the shape of a martini glass for inspiration, prepare to adopt a new food outlook—starting now.

You know the statistics—diets fail a discouraging 98 percent of the time. Those statistics aren't going to get you into a smaller pair of jeans anytime soon, are they? Could it be because so many weight loss regimes require that you follow a wacky plan that has you eating ½ cup of melon sprinkled with wheat germ and a small piece of whole grain toast every morning, the same thing for lunch, followed by an afternoon snack of warm water with a lemon wedge, and a dinner of a broiled tomato. Or perhaps you've tried diets where you have to concentrate very hard at every meal, trying desperately to remember whether it is okay to eat lots of X but not any of Y during this particular phase of the plan. Who really wants to live like that? If you are like me, you'd much rather sit down to what I had for dinner tonight—spicy fried chicken, mashed Yukon Gold potatoes, steamed broccoli, and a cold glass of white wine. And I'm thinking that a little Häagen-Dazs Dulce de Leche might be a pleasant way to finish off the evening. Care to join me? I've got an extra spoon.

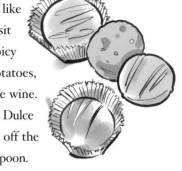

The Best Rules

The Martini Diet eating plan is relatively easy to incorporate into your life. You don't have to cut back or eliminate a whole food category, such as sugar or carbs or fat, and you don't need to focus on calories. Weight loss for the self-indulgent involves just three things:

1. **Eat Only the Very Best**
2. **Eat Somewhat Less of the Very Best**
3. **Eat the Very Best Only at Mealtimes**

Another way to think of these three rules is this—quality, quantity, and that bane of dieters: frequency.

Martini Diet Rule #1—Eat Only the Very Best

Say it out loud with me now (you'll have to put down your martini glass for a minute while you repeat this rule, because I want you to be paying very close attention): Henceforth I will eat only the very best food available. Nothing but the freshest, the finest, the very best quality food life has to offer me.

Quality? Does that strike you as an odd thing to focus on? Some strict dieters believe that they need to turn their attention away from how wonderful food is, to lose interest in food and think of food strictly as fuel to keep their bodies going. What a sad attitude. Food is not our enemy. I like to think of food as a handsome and well-bred suitor who rings the doorbell arms filled with fresh flowers and fresh shrimp, just as I am craving his presence.

Instead of losing interest in food, I want you to focus more closely than ever before on what you are eating, to enjoy every morsel, and to seek out new and varied pleasures.

The Science of Self-Indulgence

If you want to make permanent change in your weight, you really must indulge in the foods you love most. Really, you must. Marsha J. Hudnall, R.D., the nutrition director at Green Mountain at Fox Run, a women's health retreat, is a firm believer in this concept. Why? Because the minute you tell yourself you *can't* have something, you begin to obsess about it. "That increases our desire for it," she says, and when you finally do run across it you will lose all caution and control and overdo it. But if you give yourself permission to eat a modest amount of what you love most (pie, in my case!), you lessen that danger dramatically.

Slow, Slow Eating

Gourmets, food snobs, and culinary elitists have been around since the world's first dinner party. "Really, was that the freshest antelope you could club, darling? Wasn't there one with a little more marbled fat and more attractively twisted horns?" The past fifteen years has seen the rise of a new and outspoken movement dedicated to eating only the best and freshest foods, produced by only the best small farms and artisan food makers. The Slow Food movement was founded in 1986 by Carlo Petrini, an Italian man mortified by the news that a McDonald's was being built smack dab in the center of his beloved Rome. One man's culinary outrage has grown into a worldwide organization of food lovers who are horrified by the tacky fast-food life that surrounds us.

Here is an excerpt from the Slow Food Manifesto:

> *We are enslaved by speed and have succumbed to the same insidious virus: Fast Life, which disrupts our habits, pervades the privacy of our homes, and forces us to eat Fast Foods... A firm defense of quiet material pleasure is the only way to oppose the universal folly of Fast Life.*

And this is the part that makes me smile with anticipation:

> *May suitable doses of guaranteed sensual pleasure and slow, long-lasting enjoyment preserve us from the contagion of the multitude who mistake frenzy for efficiency... Our defense should begin at the table with Slow Food. Let us rediscover the flavors and savors of regional cooking and banish the degrading effects of Fast Food.*

In short, Slow Food devotees want you to sit down to a groaning table spread with platters of heirloom tomatoes, handmade breads and cheeses, some tiny new potatoes, and an aromatic and perfectly browned roast to eat with your most delightful friends, laughing and sharing for hours on end instead of rushing through yet another hurried meal of a microwaved pasta dish eaten alone in your kitchen. Who wouldn't embrace a food movement that endorses suitable doses of guaranteed sensual pleasure?

How exactly does embracing the ideas behind the Slow Food movement help you lower your weight and keep it off permanently? A most delightful friend of mine, Barbara Curtis, runs the Slow Food chapter (called Conviviums) in Lake Tahoe, California. Does she share my belief that if we eschew banal fast and processed food and vow to eat only the best it will make a big difference in our waistlines? "Absolutely. Eating as though the food mattered will definitely make a difference in your weight. If you have respect for food—and it does require respect—you will need much less of it to be satisfied. Real food, slow food, is visual; you concentrate on the way it feels in your mouth and every sense is involved. Yes, you do feel replete in a very short time. Becoming more of a food snob has kept my weight in check. Traveling on the road as a sales rep, I spent countless nights in cut-rate motels, faced with just fast-food outlets lining the streets. Rather than lower myself to eating what was available there, I would just decide the food simply wasn't good enough and wouldn't eat it. I'd rather eat a piece of fresh fruit and leave it at that than settle for a heavy, fatty meal that would leave me sorry."

Remember my earlier motto—*the higher you put your nose in the air about what you eat, the smaller your behind.* Barbara is living proof! To read more about the Slow Food movement and to find a chapter near you, check out their website at www.slowfoodusa.org.

The Science of Self-Indulgence

Dr. Arthur Agatston, the creator of the popular "South Beach Diet," confirmed my long-held belief about junk food: "The more food is preprocessed, the more fattening it will be." So an apple is better than apple juice, real oatmeal is better than instant (which has most of the fiber stripped out so that it will cook faster), and that beautiful dark brown and crusty loaf of freshly baked whole wheat bread from your local baker is a zillion times better than white bread.

Lock Up the Chemical Closet

Slow food, with its anti-fast food bedrock, will not only focus you on delicious food enjoyed with family and friends, but it will also keep you far away from two reasons our collective weight has crept up over the years—fake food and fast food.

When you begin to live steadfastly by the Martini Diet rule to **Eat Only the Very Best**, you will sidestep the fakery that surrounds us. What do I mean by fake? To begin with, don't reach for a muffin, a cookie, a drink marked "fat-free," because it isn't real food. Remember what our food goddess, Julia Child, had to say about fat-free, no-fat, or nonfat foods? That they aren't really food at all, but just "a process." On the Martini Diet you simply will not 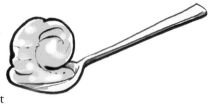 touch silly food stuffed with chemicals and all manner of ersatz ingredients. Save yourself for real food, real fat.

Once you begin to turn your nose in the air about eating preprocessed and junk food, here are just two of the unhealthy chemical bugaboos you will largely eliminate from your diet:

Trans Fats

Found naturally in meats and some dairy products, trans fats now clutter and clog up our arteries up all too frequently. They are added to most cookies, chips, and other snack foods on the supermarket shelf. Nutritionists believe that trans fats are so noxious that there really is no "safe" level for us to consume.

High Fructose Corn Syrup

In the 1980s, food manufacturers discovered that it was cheaper to use high fructose corn syrup than refined sugars in products such as soda, fruit beverages, jams, candy, cookies, and cereals, to mention just a few. What was a dollars-and-cents decision may well be the cause of the increasing obesity epidemic, though, according to the World Health Organization. The body metabolizes high fructose corn syrup differently than regular sugar, and according to the author of the book *Fatland*, we pack on the pounds faster as a result.

The Science of Self-Indulgence

Take a look at the ingredients list for this beloved product from our childhood—Filling (corn syrup, dextrose, high fructose corn syrup, water, partially hydrogenated soybean oil, corn syrup solids, sugar, crackermeal, wheat starch, modified corn starch, nonfat yogurt powder [heat-treated after culturing], dried blueberries, dried grapes, dried apples, modified wheat starch, citric acid, salt, color added, soy lecithin, natural and artificial flavor, xanthan gum, diacetyl tartaric acid esters of mono- and diglycerides, red #40 lake, blue #2 lake), enriched wheat flour, partially hydrogenated soybean oil, sugar, corn syrup, high fructose corn syrup, salt, leavening (baking soda, sodium acid pyrophosphate, monocalcium phosphate), natural and artificial flavoring, gelatin, red #40 lake, blue #2 lake, niacinamide, reduced iron, vitamin A palmitate, pyridoxine hydrocholride (vitamin B^6), riboflavin (vitamin B^2) thiamin hydrochloride (vitamin B^1) and folic acid.

What is this, chemistry class? And the calories—210, fully 50 percent of which are from fat. What is this delicious and nutritious taste treat? A blueberry fruit and yogurt Pop Tart. Think of how much happier your body would be if instead you have a piece of toasted whole wheat bread from the local baker, topped with a bit of jam you made yourself from the blueberries you and your children picked last summer.

As you may have noticed in your own life, snobs sometimes need the high-handed and dogmatic advice of other snobs in order to know just what people, places, or things we should snub and shun and feel above. To help those of you who are newly embracing food snobbery, allow me to share what I firmly believe are foods too ghastly to even consider eating. Sort of the food equivalent of Mr. Blackwell's annual Best and Worst Dressed list. Eliminate these "worst" foods from your diet immediately and much of your weight struggle will vanish without a trace.

Nine Ghastly and Tacky Types of Foods

~ **Ramen**—This looks like a simple and fast dish, but did you know those noodles are fried before they are dried? Ramen was standard fare for me when I was a young single girl. I thought it was a fairly healthy dinner to heat up a bowl of Ramen and toss in some frozen vegetables. Was I fooled. If the fat content didn't get me, the sodium would!

~ **Chicken nuggets**—I'm a mom, too, and have long assumed that letting my little boys eat chicken nuggets was a healthier alternative to a greasy burger. Turns out I was making yet another bad parenting decision. Highly processed chicken nuggets contain twice as much fat per ounce as a regular hamburger.

~ **Fast-food French fries**—The empty calories alone will pack on the pounds with this greasy treat, and the creepy thing is that French fries are pushed on us in bigger and bigger sizes. Feel superior to French fries and it will make a big difference.

~ **Crackers**—Okay, even Julia Child has admitted she eats the little fish-shaped crackers, fattening as they are. But do check the label on most commercially available crackers, they're just fat and preservatives mostly. Just stop buying them and you won't notice they are gone from your life.

~ **Frozen desserts**—Skip the entire Sara Lee and Marie Callender section of the freezer, and begin to develop a jaundiced eye when examining the dessert list at your favorite restaurant. Naively, I assumed that restaurants make most of what they offer on the menu, but after attending food industry trade shows, I've learned that is less and less true nowadays. Always ask the server whether the spectacular-sounding Chocolate Turtle Pie is made in their own restaurant kitchen, and don't be surprised if they begin to stammer.

~ **Huge muffins**—Muffins that you make yourself, straight out of the oven, are a wondrous thing. But the enormous and overly sweet commercial muffins are to be avoided under all circumstances. Big calorie and fat bombs, filled with ghastly ingredients.

~ **Anything that comes in a package of twelve or twenty-four**—really, why would you buy twelve or twenty-four of anything? Toilet paper, maybe, or perhaps AA batteries, but food? If it has enough preservatives in it to be offered in such a large shelf-stable quantity, it is simply not up to your standards. Avoiding things in these sizes will help you easily eliminate pre-packaged cookies and donuts.

~ **Anything that is jumbo or super-size**—see above. The very idea of "super-sizing" has led many of us down the path straight to obesity and unhappiness. Steer clear.

~ **Food with silly names**—The foods that you will enjoy indulging in on the Martini Diet have grown-up names such Veal Oscar, Crepes Suzette, and Steak Diane, not silly names such as Pop Tarts, Tater Tots, and Gogurt. Why would you bother eating something with a dumb name? The sillier the name, the greater the chance it is riddled with fake ingredients.

The Science of Self-Indulgence

I want you to avoid fast food joints because you are now a food snob who will eat only the best. But here is another good reason: A study of 4,000 people found that those who eat fast food at least twice a week are 50 percent more likely to be obese.

Reading books is a delightful pastime that I encourage you to pursue. Much as I want you to spend your time reading novels that will take you on exotic literary tours of the world and expand your outlook, I'd also like you to learn more about what goes on in the food world. Here are two nonfiction books that will also expand your fresh-food outlook and help you to hew to the beliefs of the Martini Diet:

~ *Fast Food Nation* by Eric Schlosser

A thoughtful and thorough examination of the health, economic, and cultural effect of the growing dominance of fast-food chains on our nation. The slaughterhouse chapter alone will keep you away from fast-food burgers forever.

~ *Fatland* by Greg Crister

The author links the cheap commercial sweetener "high fructose corn syrup" to the ever-increasing size of our countrymen. This sweetener makes food look and taste so good that it crops up in everything from soda to bread. So what's the problem? Although it tastes good, high fructose corn syrup seems to trigger fat storage.

After a two-page rant on the horrors of fake food, the question must be asked...Will I eat *anything* with trans fat or high fructose corn syrup funk? A martini-drinking girl like me won't ever qualify for sainthood. In fact, there is one thing that I know I would cross off my list if I really studied it. But since the brave and brilliant Lauren Hutton, whom I adore, once endorsed it, I'm not looking too closely at the ingredient list. My one little step back across to the dark side of food additives is... liquid diet drinks. (My personal favorite is Slim Fast, but you can find your own.) I drink the shakes; I eat the breakfast bars. I like the way they taste, and it gets that morning meal out of the way easily without too much thought or struggle. You can adopt other, healthier quickie breakfast foods—fruit, hard-boiled eggs, or high-fiber cereal. With breakfast cereals, please do read the label and choose one without high fructose corn syrup! I have the best success finding such products in the natural foods section of the grocery store.

Have I won you over to the marvels of fresh gourmet food made with real ingredients, wresting you away from the clutches of the fast, processed food demons? I do hope so. Nonscientist that I am, I've never understood where a lab-created product such as margarine came from, or why anyone would actually use it when butter itself is so darn good. Our Lady of Gin, Julia Child, says it best—"If you're afraid of butter. . . just put in cream!"

The Cheat-proof Way

Unlike most diets, where you are tempted to cheat a tiny bit one day (which as you and your swimsuit already know, leads to doing it even more the next day, and the next day. . .), the Martini Diet works. Once you have lost your taste for junk food and pre-processed food, you won't cheat at all. If you adopt the credo that only tacky people eat tacky food, why would you ever cross that line again? Think how very slim and superior you will feel from now on when you view another theatergoer from across the lobby, laden with stale popcorn dripping in fake butter spray. You would never behave like that, never.

Martini Diet Rule #2—
Eat Somewhat Less of the Very Best

Look around you on an ordinary day on an ordinary city street anywhere in the country and what will you see? Puffy bellies and big behinds, chunky arms and thick waists. The numbers are out, and they don't look good—*more than half* of American adults are overweight, and 22.3 percent are obese. What is it about our lifestyle that contributes to this sad phenomenon? Can you say the words "super-size"? Ah, of course you recognize that well-worn phrase that trips from the lips of the high school student behind the fast-food counter. But the super-size movement isn't limited to the fast-food industry. Researchers now report that portions on American plates have grown alarmingly large in restaurants and at home over the past two decades.

Why *do* we eat all this huge food? As children we were taught to clean our plates, weren't we? As well-bred adults we still have that ingrained deep down in our psyches. When that large order of fries is handed across the counter we take it on as a personal assignment—*finish this food*. When the waiter delivers an order of spareribs that overlaps the edges of the plate, we sit up straight, tie on the plastic bib, and prepare to do battle. Equally appalling is the fact that many restaurants take actual pride in the fact that they serve outlandish portions and advertise themselves accordingly. This summer a national chain of seafood restaurants has put a commercial into heavy rotation that invites viewers to come for "Endless Crab," an all-you-can-eat extravaganza. Freshly caught and cooked crab in season is a delight, particularly when my young son Julian manages to catch them in his crab ring and proudly bring the wriggling things home. But endless crab? How horrifying. Why on earth would people want to stuff themselves on it? There is indeed such a thing as too much of a good thing. We have simply lost track of what a normal serving is!

To once again place the ordinary French citizen on the ornately carved marble Martini Diet pedestal, it is worth noting that the French quite literally eat a fraction of what we do at an ordinary meal. The actual number is 75 percent. Yes, the French eat 25 percent less of everything than we do. Can you picture that scene in your mind? The thin and well-dressed Frenchwoman sits down in an atmospheric Parisian café before a modest helping of cassoulet and a bit of salad and cheese, whereas the puffy American is served a restaurant meal that is 25 percent larger. No wonder Chanel suits are cut so small.

Here we are in the twenty-first century, faced with the ever-increasing Girth of a Nation. Surely I'm not the first to make this joke (and won't be the last, I fear) or to demand that, one by one, we all need to change our eating habits and scale back the amount of food on our plates.

The fastest way to start is to put less on your plate at home, far less. Follow Rule #1 and **Eat Only the Very Best,** but take modest helpings, eat slowly and savor each bite, and then stop eating when you feel full. Once you begin to eat this way, you will be astonished at how little it really takes for you to feel full and satisfied. Don't let anyone hector you into putting more on your plate. Stand firm in the face of temptation, and your bottom will be firm, too.

A simple technique when dining out is to eat only one-third of what is on your plate. Looking closely, researchers have found that restaurant servings of fries, burgers, and soda are now two to five times larger than those in the 1970s. The seventies are quite hip these days, with Pucci dresses and halter tops everywhere. My memories of that era aren't particularly fond, but it is high time we brought back seventies-style food portions, don't you think? I wore a much smaller size then, and I'm guessing you did, too. Once again our American food goddess, Julia Child, admonishes her readers to take "a small helping. . . a little bit of everything, and it is important to have a good time eating."

Martini Measurements

If the Martini Diet Rule #2 is **Eat Somewhat Less of the Very Best**, how exactly will you know what the right amount of food is for you to slowly lose weight? Most diet plans lay out imprecise grams for just how much your serving of green vegetables should weigh, or tell you that your meat should not be bigger than your clenched fist. As you have begun to suspect, this is not that kind of diet. Instead, let's return to our martini metaphor for inspiration and guidance.

In the introduction I praised the beauty of the martini glass, so tall, so thin, so elegant. Also rather understated and small, now that I think of it. In fact, the standard martini glass holds only about 3 liquid ounces. Why not use the martini glass itself to help you judge your portions?

We've already discussed the elegant truth that, when drinking gin martinis (is there any other kind?), you must exercise restraint. One perfect martini is just enough, two might lead to trouble, and three is bound to end up in a trail of delinquent credit card bills and an unflattering picture of you in the paper.

The same elegant truth holds for food portion size. If you aren't sure just how much of something is the right amount, simply pull a clean martini glass down off the high shelf and put it to use as a measuring device. Don't overfill it please, no fair mounding your portions above the rim and smushing it in. Like a glass full of gin, your portion should be perfectly level and a respectable distance from the top of the rim. Make sure that each part of your meal fits into the glass, the whole meal doesn't have to fit! That would be tiny indeed.

So serve yourself a dollop of mashed potatoes instead of a mound, a modicum of pasta instead of a mountain, and just a modest bit of pie instead of a major slice.

For those times when a martini glass isn't available, you will have to rely on your own sophisticated sense of restraint. One egg for breakfast instead of three, the half sandwich and home-made soup special for lunches out, and very shy and restrained portions on your dinner plate.

Dessert—The Obstacle Course

Most of us can make it through the day adhering to strict diet rules, but when the sun sets and the final meal is over our willpower seems to sink as well. It is difficult to feel restrained when confronted by a slice of freshly frosted fudge brownie, isn't it?

The same rules about portion control extend to dessert as well, naturally. I can't harangue you about the size of your breakfast, lunch, and dinner, and then leave dessert out of the equation.

To stay elegantly restrained at dessert you will need to flat out ignore any kind of "recommended serving" information. Your grandmother's famed recipe for dark and caramelly Indian pudding says it serves eight; from now on, invite ten friends over to share it with you. According to the carton of Häagen-Dazs Dulce de Leche in my freezer, it contains four servings of ½ cup at 300 calories each. My method of indulging in just a spoonful or two at the end of a meal makes that same carton last and last, for two weeks on end, and adds only an extra fifty calories to my meal. Do I feel deprived? Not at all. Those few creamy bites make me feel like I'm swathed in cashmere and ready for the rest of the evening.

The Science of Self-Indulgence

The American Dietetic Association discovered through research that many unsuccessful dieters were underestimating their calories by as much as 300 percent. At the same time, these folks were overestimating their exercise!

I'll share more Martini Diet tricks on avoiding overeating in chapter six, Cinnabon Avoidance Techniques, but as long as we are talking about dessert, I will share my method of pie control. I may have already mentioned my deep and abiding love of pie once or twice or seven times before, but here is the cultural proof that pie rules—a *New York Times* editorial back in 1902 set forth the theory that pie is: *"the secret of our strength as a nation and the foundation of our national supremacy . . . no pie-eating people can ever be vanquished."* Leery as I am of supremacy claims of any kind, I'm down with this pie thing.

How do I avoid an enormous serving of berry pie that would pop the snap on my capris? Just like eating only the crispy top part of a muffin (which I know you did, too, long before there was a "Seinfeld" episode on that very technique), I eat only the top part of the crust and maybe six or seven berry-filled spoonfuls before I push it away. Yes, I know that sounds terribly wasteful, but remember what I said about learning to ignore those childhood messages about not wasting food?

The Science of Self-Indulgence

Americans eat eight billion pounds of ice cream every year. Recognizing how hard it is to resist entirely, the editors at *Prevention* magazine challenged Holly McCord, their nutrition editor, to design a diet in which they could eat ice cream every day and still lose weight. Guess what? She did it. Ice cream is a great source of calcium, and a recent study found that dieters who had high calcium intake lost more weight than dieters who had little calcium in their diets. Make no mistake, though, it was a very modest ½ cup serving.

Pie isn't the only dessert available. How would a Martini Diet devotee handle the sudden appearance of chocolate on her plate? With delight, of course. As if that handsome and well-bred suitor, food, had sensed it was just what she needed in life. I'm not suggesting chocolate is health food, but neither is it poison. Why not have a small piece of delicious dark Godiva? Just one small piece, mind you, not three or four. Every Saturday night my parents, the very slim George and Mary Alice, share one 300-calorie dark chocolate Lindt Swiss bittersweet bar between them while watching a French film. When I was younger I thought they were freakish—who can eat only half a candy bar? The older I got, the more I came to understand their approach.

I'll examine the glories of chocolate at greater length in chapter four. You will be absolutely delighted to learn that there are actual scientific reasons why you should eat it.

Living the Martini Lifestyle

 A survey by Johns Hopkins University found that 67 percent of their respondents claimed to be dieting for health reasons, and 21 percent to look better. Can we surmise that not everyone was telling the truth? I believe that looking good is certainly good for your health, so in some odd way these were honest answers.

Once you learn to control your portion size, can you include indulgent ingredients in each one of your meals? I think so. Start the day with an omelet with cheese, move on to a lunch of a small cup of creamy soup and a slice of freshly baked bread, and then have a dinner of thinly sliced red meat, grilled vegetables, and garlic mashed potatoes? Why not? Just as long as you are very clear-eyed about the size of your portions. Stick to the martini glass rule and you will see a difference on the scale.

And speaking of red meat, whatever happened to the gin? Julia Child might be signaling the waiter about now, asking about her drink, and perhaps you are, too. I fully expect you to have a glass of wine with your evening meal.

I'd recommend against it during lunch, except for those grand and special occasions that arise, and by no means should you be drinking with your oatmeal. Seriously, I believe that both liquor and wine are important parts of indulgent dining. In chapter four not only will I reveal delicious facts about why chocolate is good for you but I will also dazzle you with information about the health aspects of moderate drinking.

Martini Diet Rule #3 — Eat the Very Best Only at Mealtimes

I've devoted pages and pages to rules 1 and 2. For rule number 3, I'm going to keep it short and stern. **Eat the Very Best Only at Mealtimes** means that you have to give up eating between meals. Period. End of story. No snacking, none whatsoever. You can enjoy modest servings of luscious food of any sort three times a day, but never, ever, in between.

Let's run through the reasons snacking does not belong in your eating repertoire. First, snacking simply is not elegant. Close your eyes and try to imagine the most elegant and thin woman you know sitting down to a bag of Doritos. The late, great, Jackie Onassis? Doubt it. What about the gorgeous and poised actress Catherine Deneuve? Not likely. Or Diane von Furstenberg, who still can wear the wraparound dresses she designs? Doesn't seem right, somehow. These are not women who spend much time on the couch in front of the TV with a big bowl of crunchy snacks at their side, or drive through commuter traffic with one hand inside a paper bag of salty French fries. As a Martini Diet adherent, you will not behave in ways that are not elegant. You will rise above the common fray and reject those tacky and coarse habits, won't you?

Deciding that snacking is tacky and coarse behavior from which you will henceforth refrain (perhaps I should have worked the word "henceforth" into the subtitle of this book) will also help you keep your total food intake in the modest range. This is the second reason why you should refrain from snacking—you don't need the calories. Snacking can so easily snowball from "just a tiny taste of this" to "just a medium bag of that" and a shockingly large number of calories can be consumed in an embarrassingly short amount of time. If you don't have one cracker in between meals, then you won't run the risk of having twenty.

The Science of Self-Indulgence

In a study published in the *Journal of the American Medical Association* in 2003, researchers found that while in 1977 snacks made up 11 percent of the average American's food intake, by 1996 it had risen to 18 percent. Yet another reason for the return of the seventies.

Snacking doesn't just encompass cookies, crackers, and chips. Martini Dieters need to think about what they drink, too. Don't worry, I'm not talking about alcohol yet—I've promised you good news in chapter four. But in an earlier chapter I mentioned the stomach-turning fact that the average American consumes 150 pounds of sugar a year. Few of us are actually spooning the stuff into our mouths, so where does it all come from? Gee, maybe from soda? Along with eliminating any and all snacking, rule 3 requires that you become a soda dispenser.

The Science of Self-Indulgence

I don't care much for a full tummy at night, but there's no truth to the long-held belief that nighttime eating packs on the pounds. Some diets tell you not to eat after 7 p.m., but scientists know that a calorie is a calorie, no matter what time you consume it. So go ahead, pretend that you live in Madrid, and sit down to dinner at 10 p.m.

Dispense with soda, that is. I don't want to hurt anyone's feelings here, but drinking soda is not just a far from sophisticated thing to do—it borders on childlike. Do real grownups walk around carrying a 64-ounce wax cup of something sweet and brown and bubbly? I think not. Why not offend all my readers and add sweet coffee drinks, big cups of slushy fruit juices, and even those ubiquitous bottles of water? Civilized and sophisticated people do not walk around in public carrying a drink of anything, period. If you are thirsty, sit down in a café and order something to be consumed there at a leisurely pace. Don't wander through life slurping loudly from a paper cup.

The Science of Self-Indulgence

Does my rule about drinking in public really extend to drinking water? Not if you are running in a marathon. Go ahead and take that paper cup. And do go ahead and imbibe water in the privacy of your own office or home. Water does wonderful things for your skin, helps you feel full, and helps flush out impurities of all sorts. Don't give it up, but don't be silly about how much you need and when you need it.

Three Simple Rules

There you have it. Three simple rules make up the Martini Diet Eating Plan, rules that you will easily be able to stick to.

Martini Diet Rule #1 — Eat Only the Very Best
Martini Diet Rule #2 — Eat Somewhat Less of the Very Best
Martini Diet Rule #3 — Eat the Very Best Only at Mealtimes

You will swear off the gross and tacky food offerings that surround us in restaurants and on the grocery store shelf, saving yourself to indulge in freshly cooked food made with real ingredients instead of chemicals. You will exercise restraint when it comes to how much of this delicious food you actually eat. And you will not eat between mealtimes or wander around carrying a tacky drink in a cup.

The Martini Diet is by no means an instant way to lose weight. Once you begin to adopt these eating habits you should feel an immediate change in how full and sluggish you feel after mealtimes—you won't. Eating less during one meal will help you feel trimmer; eating less for a dozen meals will quickly show results on the scale.

By making these permanent changes in the way you live—by changing your attitudes about what food you eat and how much of it you eat—you will begin to see results on the scale. You will eat less. You will not be hungry. The slower you lose the weight, the greater the chance you will keep it off forever. You will be as sleek as a martini glass and just as refined in your approach to life.

We live in a sea of sameness in twenty-first- century America. So much of our lives are the same as the person standing next to us—most new houses look alike, our cars are so similar it is difficult to tell one from another in the parking lot, our clothes all come from the same stores, and everyone you know watches "The Sopranos" and "Sex and the City." Why would you want to eat what everyone else eats, wear what everyone else wears? Here is your chance to strike a blow for individuality and establish yourself as a person with unique tastes. It comes through in what you *won't do*—you won't "drive thru" and you won't gobble a fatty sandwich in the car while you drive to a meeting.

Once you adopt the Martini Diet Eating Plan, your memories of eating any other way will quickly fade. As Julia Child would say at the end of each of her cooking shows—*bon appetit!*

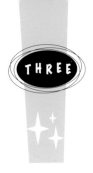

Straight Up

What was that oh-so-compelling dream life from chapter one? The luscious life in which we would lie about on satin sheets, reading novels while tuxedo-clad men surrounded us? Was that it? I've found a way you can be surrounded by tuxedo-clad men (who actually own these natty things) while getting exercise and burning fat at the same time! What could be better? Well, what about a way to exercise that increases the size of your diamonds, perhaps?

I warned you early on that indulgence does not mean indolence. Indolence, as in "an indication to laziness, that one is averse to activity, effort, or movement," to cite the actual dictionary definition. If you want to indulge your appetite for luxurious foods without further risking the size of your bottom, or if you want to indulge and lose some of the weight you have now, you will need to develop the mindset that exercise can also be an indulgent way to spend your time. Most of us do not think of exercise as particularly indulgent, I'll grant you that. The first image that springs to mind when we hear the word exercise is often that of a sweaty, red, grimacing face, clenched in distaste as we try to do just one more situp, just one more knee bend, just one last lap around the indoor track. Perhaps there should be other images then, more appealing mental images, such as that of a straight-backed rider in a black velvet jacket taking a horse over a jump, an elegant woman gliding alone through the water in a seamless breaststroke, a lithe leotard-clad dancer flexing before the barre, or a brave and sharp-witted fencer lunging toward her opponent. Is exercise beginning to sound a weensy bit more appealing to you now?

The bottom line about exercise is that your body needs it. Regardless of the state of your health, you *need* to move. You need exercise to maintain the weight you have now or to lose excess weight, to stay limber and supple as you age, to build bones and strength and prevent ordinary injuries. Rather than avoid working up a sweat entirely, the more indulgent attitude is to find something you enjoy that will become an integral part of your life. An activity that enhances your life and becomes a delightful addition to your day, rather than a chore that you must suffer through. Even if you have never before made any kind of exercise a part of your life, even if you have shunned the idea entirely, I believe that you will be drawn to at least one of the indulgent forms I will tempt you with here.

As with the rest of the Martini Diet lifestyle, you need to embrace the idea that your time is valuable, and that (let's add one of my grand-sounding *henceforths* here) henceforth you will spend it doing only what you enjoy. You have vowed to make the switch to eating only wonderful food (in delicate servings), to turning your back on the mundane and inelegant and turning your nose up at the many culinary things that simply aren't good enough for you. With all of that free time you have, now that you are no longer snacking in the afternoons or running out for a smoothie, you will be able to devote yourself to further transforming your body.

When it comes to exercise, feel free to turn up your nose at much of what other people do, too. Sweat like a pig in a hot room full of people, turning and twisting your body in all manner of contortions? Awfully common, don't you think? Just a tad too popular to really interest you, who is dedicated to carving your own elegant swath through life. Be stretched and pulled by medieval-looking machines, regardless of the wondrous claims their adherents make? Again, so terribly ordinary.

The Science of Self-Indulgence

About 45 percent of women and 25 percent of men are trying to lose weight at any one time, but only one-fifth of those folks are actually trying to do it through a combo of fewer calories and more exercise! The rest are, what, using voodoo?

I'll spare you an exact repeat of my soapbox speech in the first chapter. As you may recall, it had something to do with the unrealistic images of women's bodies that swarm around us in the media, making us all feel far less than perfect. Just as our feelings about how much we need to weigh are influenced by glossy magazine photos of superthin models, our feelings about just what our body parts should look like are equally influenced. Thin, toned upper arms are a must. Taut thighs the size of young willow trees are the only ones acceptable in public, and stomachs should be as slim and flat as possible. If you can't achieve that look—why bother? Bring on the chocolate mousse and settle back on the couch. Now, now, that is not the Martini Diet attitude!

Instead, have a more realistic ideal for how your body will look. Proud as I am of the fifty stomach crunches I try to do each day, I read once that the routine of a well-known model is to do *500* a day. Ah, a mere difference of 450. Her body is her *job*, and doing 500 situps is what keeps her working. My body is definitely not *my* job, so why bother to compare myself to the professionals? Even armed with that information it is hard to look at a picture of a tiny tummy and not feel like I am falling behind.

Speaking of behinds, understand that even professional athletes sometimes have a bit of jiggle and give. One of my long laundry list of ex-boyfriends came with unlimited access to courtside seats at a major arena. Sometimes it was disconcerting to sit so close (the sight of a herd of professional basketball players headed your way is terrifying), but sometimes it gave me the opportunity to see the unexpected. My heart soared once while watching an exhibition tennis match featuring Martina Navratilova. Yes, certainly her strength and artistry thrilled me, but so too did the fact that when her skirt rode up as she served I saw a teensy bit of cellulite on her thighs. Thank you, God.

So, why not try this while adopting the Martini lifestyle—instead of desiring a 24-inch waist, make achieving a strong, toned, and healthy body your goal. Not only can it be achieved, but it may well get you farther in life than a tiny waist will.

When it comes to exercise, what, then, can be considered indulgent? I am attracted to the kinds of sports and activities that somehow conspire to make you look good while performing them or that have really wonderful wardrobes to go along with them. Let's look closely at a few of them here...

The Science of Self-Indulgence

Don't just sit there, move! If you are more likely to be found on the couch in front of the TV instead of out on the dance floor, heed this—researchers at the Harvard School of Public Health have confirmed that TV watching is strongly linked to weight gain. Not only are you just sitting there without burning calories, but you are also being subjected to all those junk food ads that encourage you to eat and eat.

Women and Their Horses

I loved horses when I was ten, did you? Oh, how I begged my parents for a horse, any horse, even a small one would do. Alas, no horse ever showed up Christmas morning on my lawn, but that didn't keep me from climbing aboard, as an adult. At last I could control a sweaty beast with just my leg muscles—what could be better?

It was a world of elegant horsewomen that I was longing for, not the John Wayne world of big Western saddles. After living a few years in my horsey northern California suburb, I finally tired of jealously eyeing the bold women I would sometimes see in the grocery store, their sleek riding pants and trim leather boots trailing dust behind them. Heavens, their butts looked small in those pants! Do only trim women ride, I wondered, or does riding make them look that good in those elegant pants? I signed up for private lessons, daydreaming of the day I, too, would wander casually around the grocery store, looking like Jackie O just in from a hunt.

In fact, riding with an English saddle does indeed have a beneficial effect on how we look in pants. "I was voted 'best butt' at my television station for several years running," my friend Sue Atkinson confessed, harkening back to an innocent time when it was perfectly okay to think about your coworkers behinds. Sue began riding at age seven, and at age fifty-six has extraordinary legs and a bottom that still looks trim in tight pants. Why? Because an English saddle requires you to "post" up and down as the horse moves, essentially performing an endless series of ballet pliés, lifting your upper body over and over from the just the balls of your feet balanced on the stirrups. Try it and see how those leg and thigh muscles work. My first lessons were followed by generous amounts of Motrin.

My editor, Paula Munier, the very woman whose lament about the size of her inner princess' behind inspired me to write *The Martini Diet,* has also recently returned to the stable after an absence of a decade or two. "Not only does your behind get worked while riding, but if you also curry and brush the horse afterwards, as most stables require, you will get a pretty good upper body workout too." My friend Sue also points out that, if you own your own

The Science of Self-Indulgence

Riding looks so very *Town & Country*, so how could you be burning calories? Posting at a trot for an hour burns 420 calories, and you may not be able to walk the next day because your legs get such a workout. Grooming a horse (which you will probably have to do even if you don't own one, as most riding schools expect you to groom and saddle your own horse) for an hour burns another 525 calories.

horse, you will spend quite a bit of time hauling big bales of hay and big shovels of... well, use your imagination. Yet another way to get a workout.

Is riding just a rich woman's sport? It certainly can be expensive, of course, if you own a horse and assume all the expenses that go along with it. Riding a few days a week at a stable on a horse you don't own is not an outrageous expense, though. My private lessons are $35 each; when I join a group lesson, it costs less. Yes, that is more expensive than jumping around in a gym studio crowded with girls in leotards, but not out of the question.

The Science of Self-Indulgence

So, on the Martini Diet, can you exercise and drink at the same time? No, please don't. For one thing, you don't want to risk your crystal glasses near the pool, stable, or ice rink! And even after you've finished your ride, run, dance, or swim, you need to give your body a rest before you indulge in alcohol. Drink plain water first instead, or your dehydrated body will use whatever you're drinking to replenish what you sweated out. Water is better than gin for that task!

They're Playing Your Song

What was that I promised earlier about well-dressed men and exercise? One of the most elegant, and most athletic, ways to exercise in an indulgent fashion is ballroom dancing.

A dear friend of mine had the great good fortune to marry a Swedish count. As if that weren't glossy enough, the count is also a good dancer. They met and bonded on the dance floor, and it has played a large role in their married life ever since. "I spend as much time on the dance floor as I can each week," she told me, "and it is just as much exercise as going to the gym. Dancing works every muscle in your body, believe me." In fact, next to swimming, movement experts say that dancing is the best exercise there is.

Once again, a way to both move your body and wear cool clothes. Can you imagine how much happier you will be gliding around a polished wooden ballroom floor in a floating chiffon dress than doing situps and pushups in a pair of old sweat pants? "Here is how I would sum up the difference between working out at the gym, and spending an hour or two dancing," the countess told me. "It is the difference between having a picnic and dining with the queen." Guess which one is closer to dining with the queen?

Countess Beth now has her own ballroom to dance in (he is such a sweet man, that count), but where will you be able to take a spin around the floor? Every city has dance studios that would love to see you as a student, either with a partner or alone. Community colleges and adult learning organizations such as The Learning Annex are also a good place to find both classes and a place to dance. If you don't already have a partner in the dance of life, this may well be a way to find one...

Just as physical as ballroom dancing and a good deal sexier is salsa and tango dancing. You can picture tango dancing, can't you? Two stylish and impeccably dressed people with their cheeks pressed together, faces forward and arms stretched out, as they parade across the floor to a Latin beat. "It feels as good as it looks," said one dance instructor as he stood on the edge of the polished dance floor watching a sinuous couple float by.

You needn't dedicate your life to the dance to see a physical effect. Because dancing is so physical and can burn so many calories (396 an hour), just signing up for classes two nights a week will make a big difference. "I have been ballroom dancing for some thirty years now, and it has absolutely made a difference in my body," the countess said. "My personal trainer is always astonished at how strong and slim my legs are. It is all from dancing, and in high heels, no less!"

Swan Lake

The velvet curtain lifts, and as the sound of violins fills the air, you walk gracefully out to center stage in a pink tulle skirt. Rising up on your toe shoes, you take your first delicate steps toward the audience and begin the familiar dance of the dying swan.

As a gawky teen, I felt like a dying swan in ballet class and dropped out early. What about you? Did you hang in there and learn every last position and attitude? It isn't too late to take it up again as an indulgent exercise form. An actual ballet class provides an all-around exercise workout and is far more stimulating than an aerobics class done to a steady hip hop beat. "Dancing is dreaming," a committed ballerina once told me, and by taking ballet classes once again as an adult you will find it is never too late to dream.

Whereas ballroom dancing is an activity geared to grown-ups, most ballet schools cater to the tiny girl set. Don't let the fear of stepping on small children keep you away from the barre, though. Many ballet schools do have classes that are for adults, and everyone there will feel just as lumpy and awkward as you do at first.

If you are too reluctant to be seen in public in a leotard, there is still a lovely way to give your body the incredible benefits of ballet. The New York City Ballet has two different one-hour workouts available on video and DVD. Narrated by the ballet master in chief, Peter Martins, this routine is remarkably easy to follow (even for those of us who quit at fourteen). Starting with warm-up stretches and moving through ab exercises and then to a long series of *pliés,* this tape really gives you a thorough workout and leaves you feeling long and lean. I love the abdominal exercises done to the soundtrack of chamber music (the dancer parts do use real ballet music, though) and the somber voice of the ballet master intoning, "Strong abs are not only appealing to the eye, but they act as a support to the entire body." Yes, of course. And your pants fit better, too.

Even if you can't track down this or any other ballet workout tape, you can still involve ballet moves in your own exercise routine. When traveling, I always do *pliés,* in my hotel room to help combat thigh jiggle. You can picture a *plié,* can't you? Just a fancy name for a knee bend, really. But when you are channeling your inner ballerina and imagining that you are warming up behind the velvet curtain, about to make your debut on the stage, it adds a bit of glamour and romance to an ordinary movement.

Exercise in High Heels

Public ice skating rinks are regularly flooded after a Winter Olympics, filled with young girls hoping to be just like Sarah Hughes. Skating in and around the groups of girls you will also see full-grown women, though, gliding past and hoping to be mistaken for a slightly more mature ice queen, such as Katerina Witt. "Not just a professional skater like Katerina Witt, but you can also feel a bit like a Vegas showgirl in some of those sequin outifts," Caroline Benard tells me. At forty, Caroline returned to the rink not only to get in shape but also to spend a few hours a week being taller. Yes, taller. "For anyone who dreamed of having long legs, just put on a pair of ice skates and you'll instantly grow 3 inches!" Perfect for a Jimmy Choo devotee like me, ice skating can feel like exercising in high heels. You are not only instantly taller, but you also feel elegant and (once you master the basics and can stay on your feet) graceful, too. Not a feeling you are likely to get from a long jog through the woods, is it?

While skating, you will be so focused on learning the moves and improving your balance that it really won't feel like exercise at all (until the next morning, when you ease yourself out of bed). At the rink Caroline visits several times a week there is a group of women who have not only mastered the basics of skating but are also now moving on to learning ice dancing. Dressed in flowing skirts and tops decorated with healthy dollops of sequins and glitter, perhaps they, too, are hoping to be mistaken for Katerina Witt.

If you plan to ice skate as your indulgent form of exercise, I would recommend starting out with just one session a week and building up from there. It will take a few months for your body to build up the strength and suppleness to skate several times a week, but when you do reach that level, you will be delighted by the leg muscles you have developed in the process.

En Garde!

Have you ever been so frustrated with someone in your life, so very fed up with him, that you just wanted to whack him on the head? Or point a menacing-looking sword toward her and slowly advance in a threatening way? Women who fence can do just that! Here is your chance to engage in an elegant exercise and work out your bottled-up anger at the same time.

"As a form of exercise, fencing is sneakily aerobic," Mary Griffith, of the Sacramento Fencing Club, told me. And she would know, as her other forms of exercise include writing books and fixing computers. Both of Mary's daughters have been competitive fencers, and her younger daughter recently confessed that the occasional head-whacking part was what held her attraction.

Fencing is an intricate and graceful martial art, one of the original Olympic sports. Although it tends to have a more European flair, the U.S. Olympic fencing team is the reigning champion. A challenge to both your body and your mind in a way that most sports are not, it is a game that rewards mental agility over sheer strength and power. What does that mean to you? That if you learn how to fence you can beat up the guys.

You've seen pirate movies, so I know you can picture fencing in your mind. Two guys in puffy shirts waving swords at each other and lunging forward before shuffling backward to avoid the opponent's sword. Much of fencing is done from that same bent-knee, slightly squatting position, the same *plié* position I keep touting with ballet and horseback riding! While fencing, dancing, or riding an English saddle, your leg and thigh muscles are constantly being worked in that semi-bent position. While semi-crouched in that position, you advance forward and backward, forward and backward again and again, while at the same time controlling your foil and holding one arm gracefully back over your head. It really is a beautiful sport to watch, and a remarkably physical one to engage in.

Do women really fence? My college roommate (at a genteel women's college, no less) was an avid fencer who spent hours parrying and riposting. Sure, fighting with swords seems a bit scary, but fencing is actually quite safe. The U.S. Fencing Association claims you are more likely to be injured jogging than fencing.

Fencing is not a sport you can just take up on your own. You will need to find a fencing academy or club in your area. Even though the foils and sabres are tipped so that they don't actually cut, you still don't want to pick one up and wave it around without someone telling you how. And the exercise aspect comes from both the warm-ups that fencing students undergo before they begin to fight and the matches themselves. Like riding jodhpurs, fencing knickers are more form-fitting than baggy sweatpants. And as with riding, the more you fence, the better you will look in those pants!

A Short Walk in the Country

Everywhere you look, in my neighborhood and in yours, too, I'm guessing, someone is out for a walk and looking very determined to lose weight doing it. You can tell from the look on her face and the way she pumps up her arms with such great purpose. Many of these folks have hit the pavement due to the recently announced target fitness mark of 10,000 steps a day.

Ten thousand steps a day... how is it possible to do that without fainting from boredom?

In this chapter, I've tried to focus on exercises that have a bit more panache and élan to them, not your run-of-the mill sort of pastime. But with all of America out walking, should we not join and see how it works?

Just how far do you have to walk to keep your jeans loose, I wondered? Images of an elegantly thin and straight-backed Jackie O walking daily at the reservoir at Central Park came to mind, and wasn't Greta Garbo also a well-known walker? I cling to small scraps of glamour in an effort to escape the suburban image of walking for exercise, you see.

Walking to get somewhere, on the other hand, also seems more urbane and glamorous than what those of us marching down the road in sports bras and sweatpants are doing. Instead of tramping through the early morning light to shed weight, perhaps instead I am gliding through the streets of Paris on my way home from a late-night tryst. French women also spend their days walking around picking up a little of this, a little of that, some cheese at this shop, some bread at that one. Goodness, I have such Paris envy, does it come through that clearly in this book?

But enough about the French. Here at home we need to get our spreading behinds out of our cars and back to doing what nature intended, helping us get from one place to the other. Urban planners are now pointing toward suburban sprawl as just one more reason for America's weight problem; communities that are set up for cars and lack sidewalks seem to breed large people who live unhealthy sedentary lifestyles.

The Science of Self-Indulgence

Every talk show and magazine article is touting the goal of walking 10,000 steps a day. Just how far is that, anyway? Depending on the length of your stride, about 4½ miles. And how many calories will you burn? If you walk for thirty minutes at a pace of 4 miles an hour, you will burn 165 calories, 225 if you are on a slight incline, and a whopping 360 if you are walking up a 10-percent incline. Double that when you walk for an entire hour. But when you turn around and walk back down that incline to get home, your calorie burn rate will, alas, drop.

For a shocking look into your life and habits, I recommend you purchase a pedometer. Sure, you could just count quietly to yourself as you walk, but walking with your lips moving makes you look like a crazy person and your neighbors might think about calling the police. Avoid possible arrest and instead spend the stunning sum of $12 (I bought mine at Target; check out the sports department) for a pedometer you can hook to your belt and wear everywhere throughout the course of your day.

Once you begin wearing a pedometer, it becomes a huge challenge. *How many steps did I walk today,* I wonder as I glance down. And if the number just doesn't seem big enough for that time of day I just do a short bit of dancing to get moving and inch that number up. Yes, if the neighbors spotted my dancing it might look just as nutty as walking down the street counting to myself. At least I'm dancing on my own property, anyway.

And does it have an effect, all this pedestrian walking? In fact it does. Starting your day with a short fast walk around your neighborhood is a great way to get the blood pumping. I know that even if you take up fencing or ballroom dancing or ice skating you won't be able just to roll out of bed in the morning and do those things. A brisk walk, on the other hand, is possible on the spur of the moment.

How can we make walking luxurious or indulgent? Wearing high heels isn't going to work with this one, and I don't want to see you out on the street in your finest evening clothes. What we can do, though, is walk in luxurious places. On the beaches of Hawaii. Down the streets of Paris. Over the hills of Tuscany. Plan vacations in places where you can walk and walk, and the more you walk on vacation the more you will look forward to doing it in your everyday life.

Merrily We Swim Along

Do you ever crave solitude? I know I do. So many of my waking moments are accompanied by the shrill sound of someone calling "Mamaaaaa," or an endlessly ringing phone, or a steady stream of visitors through the office. Like Garbo, I VANT to be alone. And in these moments I close my eyes and picture an unbroken surface of cool blue water, just waiting for me to dive into the center. If you are tired of those crowded workout classes and long for a quiet and unhurried way to move your body, my dears, then I recommend you take up the zenlike experience of swimming laps alone with your thoughts and your dreams.

Although most of us think of the Australian crawl stroke when we picture swimming laps, I am firmly in favor of the more sedate breaststroke. Swimming breaststroke not only looks elegant and keeps your hair from drying out and your eyes open for tiny children treading water in your path, but—listen to this, ladies—it also makes your diamonds look HUGE. As you swim languid stroke after stroke, do take the time to admire how large and sparkly diamonds look when the sunlight hits them underwater. Any diamonds, big or small. Imagine a DeBeers commercial starring you, listen to the stirring violins they use as their corporate image music, and hear it in your head as you swim forth.

Unlike so many high-intensity sports that seem better suited to the youthful, swimming is a sport for all ages. I have a delightful friend in Hawaii, Kaimuki, who at age eighty-five still swims daily at a private club in Honolulu. She works her thirty laps a day into a full schedule of regular tennis matches and surfing. Online surfing, that is, a newly acquired passion.

While growing up in San Francisco, Kaimuki told me, "My father thought I was too much of a tomboy and that swimming was a ladylike sport that would be suitable," she laughed. "It is a dull sport compared to the action in tennis, but nothing beats the beauty of swimming outdoors, looking up at the sky." Whereas I prefer to swim my laps breaststroke, Kaimuki is fond of backstroke, which gives her plenty of opportunity to skywatch. After spending so much of her time in a bathing suit she still looks trim. "Oh, I'm vain. When you know you will be seen in public in a bathing suit you make a real effort to keep your stomach down!" I'll return again to the puzzle of my Jodhpurs Theory—most women who wear them look good in them, but is it from the riding or because they make the effort to look good in tight pants they wear in public? A chicken and egg conundrum.

The Science of Self-Indulgence

How many calories will we burn in the pool? An incredible 720 an hour, but who is really going to swim for an hour? Not me. Instead, I set an exercise goal of twenty laps and blithely assume it is doing remarkable things for my middle-aged bust and thighs.

If you are self-conscious about how you look in a bathing suit, do not despair. You need only blush for the nanosecond it will take for you to drop your robe on a chaise and leap quickly into the pool. It will be a painless process, I promise. Please be gentle on yourself when assessing your bathing suit suitability; remember that you are a real woman with a real woman's body. The more time you spend in the pool the more comfortable you will be in a suit and, of course, the greater the benefit to your body. For a sweatless good time, I highly recommend it!

Indulge in Exercise Daily

Have you sensed a theme in the exercises I've highlighted here? Perhaps the theme of... fantasy? Or at the very least, the desire to recapture your own girlhood fantasy about the way your life would be as a grown-up girl? I wanted a horse and shiny leather boots and no one would ever permit it. I fantasized about growing up to be a ballerina, but then never stuck to the classes. What about you? Does the idea of gliding effortlessly around a ballroom floor stir some earlier longing for a way of life you may have dreamed of to get through math class? Here is your chance to make the kind of life you wanted, to indulge in the kinds of interests that attracted your younger, less realistic self!

There is a second theme that runs through these sports—that of good posture and standing tall. Ballet, fencing, riding, dancing, all of these will make you stand like a strong and elegantly powerful woman who faces life with an amused smile. Not only will your body be transformed by these indulgent exercises, but your outlook will be, too. Picture your newly elegant stance as you stand there in the moonlight, poised in a black lace cocktail dress, raising a thin martini glass to your ruby lips.

Can you see that image clearly in your mind? I want you to hold on to it as you become an active and involved woman who bounds out of bed every morning ready to indulge. Martini Diet enthusiasts don't think of exercise as a chore to be struggled through a few times a week. They choose activities they enjoy, activities that will bring them into contact with fascinating people and expand their horizons. What are *you* waiting for?

The Science of Self-Indulgence

A long-term study conducted by Johns Hopkins found that men who played tennis as young boys were far more likely to still be playing regularly as adults than boys who played basketball. One of my favorite artists, Wayne Thiebaud, plays several times a week at the spry age of eighty-four. Like trying to decide which came first—the body and the confidence to wear jodhpurs in public, or the ability to look good in jodhpurs because you ride several times a week—do eighty-four year olds play tennis and swim because they are active and healthy, or are they active and healthy because they play?

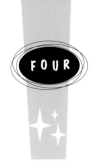

FOUR

Candy Is Dandy, But Liquor Is Quicker (And Fat Is Fine)

Ogden Nash, who actually did write the little ditty about how candy is dandy but liquor is quicker, also wrote this lovely ode to a martini:

A DRINK WITH SOMETHING IN IT

There is something about a martini,
A tingle remarkably pleasant;
A yellow, a mellow martini;

I wish I had one at present.
There is something about a martini,
Ere the dining and drinking begin,
And to tell you the truth,
It is not the vermouth—
I think perhaps it is the gin.

As you know, I am not a scientist. But that hasn't prevented me from closely following the most exciting scientific developments since we landed a man on the moon or figured out how two people can share one mattress with two different types of firmness. I have thick and important-looking files filled with clippings and articles about three of my favorite topics and the latest medical information on them. Who wouldn't be interested in the science behind chocolate, liquor, and fat?

In an earlier chapter, I perched on a soapbox to lecture you gently (I hope it was gentle, anyway) about unrealistic body images women receive from the media. Instead of a soapbox, with this lecture I'll stand in front of a chalkboard to give you a bit of a food-science talk. Or feel free to picture me in a natty business suit, standing in a gleaming mahogany conference room giving a masterful PowerPoint presentation on this topic. As I'm talking about the glories of chocolate, liquor, and fat, I guarantee it will be a damn sight more interesting than the last PowerPoint presentation you suffered through.

Chocolate, once the bane and bugaboo of dieters everywhere, has been reborn in the twenty-first century as a food that is positively good for us. That one fact is enough to end any nostalgic yearning for days gone by, isn't it? Whereas in the creaky olden days of dieting chocolate came under scrutiny for its caloric and fat content, it is now celebrated for a whole host of healthful attributes. Let's take a deeper look at the science that justifies elevating our beloved chocolate to "good-for-you" status.

The Mood-Boosting Chemicals

Chocolate makes you feel good. You and I have both known that for years. But what is it in chocolate that makes us feel so good?

~ **Caffeine and Theobromine**—Caffeine in your coffee gives your day a nice kick, but the typical chocolate bar has only one-tenth of the caffeine in a cup of regular coffee. Theobromine is also a mild stimulant, though, and working together, these two give you a mood boost.

~ **Phenylethylamine**—You know that incredible high you get when you are first falling in love? You thought it was simply the sight of your tall, blond, and hunky lover, but in fact it is a brain chemical called phenylethylamine. That this same chemical is also found in chocolate proves, I think, that life is indeed perfect.

~ **N-acylethanolamines**—According to *Family Circle* magazine, these compounds can mimic the effects of a fatty acid found in marijuana. Groovy. No wonder we crave chocolate at such weird times.

Healthful Compounds (Oh Joy!)

Not only does chocolate naturally contain the mood-boosting chemicals listed above, but eating chocolate also has these actual health benefits.

~ **Flavonoids**—Flavonoids are powerful antioxidants, compounds that protect against health problems by defending your body against free radicals, which are thought to trigger cancer, stroke, and heart disease. Studies have shown that people with high levels of flavonoids in their blood also have a much lower risk of suffering from lung cancer, asthma, type 2 diabetes, and prostate cancer. You can find flavonoids in some fruits and vegetables, such as strawberries and garlic, but chocolate is a richer source of certain flavonoids than those traditionally healthy items. Who knew?

~ **Cocoa butter**—We'll look more closely at fat itself at the end of this chapter, but the fat found in chocolate, the cocoa butter that gives chocolate such a creamy texture on your tongue, is rich in both stearic acid and oleic acid, two kinds of benign fats. Cocoa butter is also rich in some other types of saturated and polyunsaturated fats.

~ **Copper and magnesium**—These two minerals are known to help keep hearts healthy, and chocolate is a good source of both. Magnesium is critical for keeping our bones strong and our teeth healthy. Just before our period starts, we ladies have lower magnesium levels, which could be why we crave chocolate right about then. Eat a bit and don't feel guilty.

The Science of Self-Indulgence

While we are dancing and twirling in the air over the good news about chocolate, it is important to remember that any food high in fat and sugar will put on the pounds if you overindulge. Remember the Martini Diet watchwords—restrained and refined. Be on your best refined and restrained behavior and don't take this news as an excuse to eat from one end of the chocolate aisle to the next. As with martinis, one is enough. One small helping of dark chocolate, please not two or three or four.

Extraordinary, isn't it? That something so reviled by the food police should turn out to be wonderful for your health. Perhaps the day is not far off when scientists reveal that wearing very high heels and red nail polish prevents most disease. Until then I will keep scanning the science section of the newspaper with bated breath.

The Science of Self-Indulgence

All of these marvelous properties are found in dark chocolate, and Dove Dark is the most often cited as a good source of all of chocolate's best attributes. Dove Dark was actually used in a study at U.C. Davis to test the reputed heart-healthy benefits. Researchers gave the volunteers 1⅓ ounces of Dove Dark and found that it reduced LDL oxidation and boosted antioxidant levels and HDL concentrations in the blood. Another reason to read the science section of the newspaper—perhaps another study will be announced and they will need more volunteers!

How to Eat Chocolate

What, now that there is actual science behind the benefits of eating chocolate there also have to be instructions? No, of course not. This being the Martini Diet, geared toward weight loss for the self-indulgent, though, I think it is important to apply the brakes a bit here in our narrative. Remember our three basic rules of eating on the Martini Diet? Sure you do, they're so easy. The first one is to **Eat Only the Very Best**. Then we simply **Eat Somewhat Less of the Very Best**. And finally, we **Eat the Very Best Only at Mealtimes**. How then, do we safely add chocolate to our plan without reversing all that we've accomplished? Slowly, slowly, my dears.

We eat only the very best chocolate because it is only the very best, the very darkest and richest and most European chocolate that contains all these delightful properties. Drinking a chocolate shake from a fast-food joint is not going to do your health or your body any good, nor is a series of quickly consumed milk chocolate candy bars that you grabbed from the rack next to the checkout counter. Put those back *now*.

Instead, we might do well to emulate my own thin parents, George and Mary Alice. In chapter 2, I shared their decades-long Saturday night habit of splitting a Swiss chocolate bar (while watching a French film, or sometimes a Swedish one). Healthy, thin, and still quite chic in their seventies, they have been doing their own type of research every weekend, haven't they?

And we eat only modest amounts of the very best chocolate at mealtime, don't we? Even though it is now revealed as a superb source of various and sundry good things, that is no reason to indulge in it mid-morning or late afternoon. Save your chocolate indulgence for the evening, and have a small piece with a glass of red wine after dinner. As you'll read in a minute or two, that delicious combo is even healthier!

Living the Martini Lifestyle

 Now that Old Europe is morphing into one big family, is chocolate in danger? Christian Constant, a French chocolate maker, believes it is. Due to the newly enacted EU standards, up to 5 percent of the cocoa butter in chocolate may now be replaced with other, cheaper types of fats and still be called "chocolate." "If chocolate, then why not 5 percent vegetable fat in butter?" he asks, "Or wine? It's sad, because we're assuring a move toward a more synthetic world, in all domains."

Chocolate Milk?

After all this talk about darkly delicious chocolate, a big cold glass of milk sounds perfect, doesn't it? Actually, no, it wouldn't be perfect, and here's why: Despite the fact that we all know calcium is a good thing for our little feminine bones, European researchers say that drinking milk while eating dark chocolate somehow discourages the body's ability to absorb the protective compounds in chocolate. And the reason that milk chocolate isn't nearly as full of healthy things compared to dark chocolate is the simple fact that milk chocolate *has only half as much actual chocolate* as dark chocolate. Ah.

Liquor Is Quicker

Now that we have assured ourselves that an ounce or two of deep, dark chocolate is a sturdy part of the staff of life, let's get down to the drinking. Why would a book called *The Martini Diet* actually wait three or four chapters to discuss martinis? Because, my dears, they are so very worth waiting for. Practice patience in life; it is a virtue that comes in handy in so many ways, whether you are waiting for the call from Hermes to say your Birken bag has arrived or waiting for the bartender to notice that your glass is empty. Your patience is about to be rewarded.

As you have repeatedly heard, I am fond of a martini or two. In fact, I wanted to call this book *Drink More Gin*, but my publisher objected. Where did all this blatant martini-worship come from? It comes from growing up in a household where the adults considered their cocktail hour to be sacrosanct, not to be intruded upon by noisy children or pesky phone calls. Those glasses of gin reigned supreme in the Basye household. Martinis are, as

E. B. White, famed *New Yorker* writer and author of children's classics *Charlotte's Web* and *Stuart Little*, put it, "the elixir of quietude."

How did my parents know that gin would turn out to be a welcome part of a healthy diet decades later? Ah, they always were more sophisticated than the world around them. Not only does gin indeed turn out to be healthy, but so too does Scotch, bourbon, rum, and vodka.

A welcome headline in *Newsweek* early in 2003 was the following: "Rx: Two Martinis a Day—Researchers say regular drinking lowers men's risk of heart attack." Raise your glasses, fellow martini fans, science is on our side. What did these delightful researchers discover? In a study published in the *New England Journal of Medicine*, Harvard researchers documented that men who imbibed in regular, moderate consumption of beer, wine, and hard liquor cut their risk of a heart attack by one-third. And women, do we just have to sit there and watch them drink? Although we can safely consume less alcohol than men (because our bodies react differently to alcohol), some nice British researchers released a study in 2000 that showed one glass of wine a day did the trick.

Living the Martini Lifestyle

 Interior designer Katherine Stephens shared this advice with the readers of *Architectural Digest:* "A friend once told me that the secret to good decorating is just to fill your rooms with liquor and friends." Sounds like a good policy to me.

What is it about liquor that can actually lower our risk of heart disease? All kinds of alcohol raise our levels of HDL, the so-called "good cholesterol," and lower our levels of a blood-clotting protein. The anticoagulant qualities in liquor are similar to those of a daily dose of aspirin (and taste much better, too).

Where does hard liquor fit in with a weight-loss program, though? When observing Rule #2, **Eat Somewhat Less of the Very Best**, I'm afraid that we will have to drink somewhat less as well. Liquor is by no means calorie-free, not even the deceptively clear ones such as gin and vodka. You may have noticed that this is the very first time the concept of "calories" has reared its fuzzy head here in this diet book, and I am only mentioning it here in an offhand way. I don't want you to be consumed with counting calories; I want you to **Eat and Drink the Very Best Available** (Rule #1) while observing Rule #2. So it behooves you to be aware of what you are drinking so that if your scale doesn't go down fast enough after changing your eating habits you will examine your drinking habits.

The Science of Self-Indulgence

Drinking liquor may also be good for your mind as well as your body. Researchers at Boston's Beth Israel Deaconess Medical Center discovered that adults aged sixty-five and older who drank one to six glasses of alcohol a week had a 30 percent lower risk of developing dementia than those who did not drink at all.

Calories in Liquor

Red, white, and rosé wines are all in the same 21 calories-per-ounce range. That means if you have a standard glass of wine (3.5 ounces), you are in the 75 calorie range. Friends who pour big glasses of wine at parties are pouring closer to 100 calories into your glass.

Gin, vodka, rum, scotch, and bourbon are higher in calories than wine, about 64 calories per ounce. I do hope, though, that you aren't drinking much more than one drink. When living the Martini lifestyle, we seek to be refined and restrained in all things, and drinking is one of them.

Those tacky but popular mixed fruity drinks are, as you may have guessed, higher in calories than just straight liquor. A piña colada is loaded with sugar and 6 grams of fat; you might as well eat cheesecake instead. I've been stern about this before: Drink like a grown-up. Grown-ups like the taste of liquor; they don't doctor it up with silly fruit juices.

Now that I've worked so hard to celebrate drinking liquor as part of a healthy diet, do I need to sound a cautionary note about alcohol abuse? Judging from the ghastly drinking and driving records it would seem that many of us do need to be reminded that liquor requires responsible behavior. Drinking and driving play no part in the Martini Diet lifestyle; it is simply not done. A martini is an adult drink, as are all types of liquor and wine. So act like an adult when you drink. An adult doesn't binge and doesn't go overboard. Should you find that your one moderate glass of vodka on the rocks or small batch bourbon seems to morph into three or four on a nightly basis, please stop and get help.

In Vino Veritas — In Wine There Is Truth

The best-fed and most sophisticated of our Founding Fathers, Thomas Jefferson, believed that "good wine is a necessity of life." Not surprisingly, Mr. Jefferson spent many years living in

Living the Martini Lifestyle

 Drinking martinis has sometimes been described as a pastime of the privileged, an image that I am happy to promote. As the author of *Wear More Cashmere*, a book that encourages readers to pamper themselves with great frequency, and a devoted martini drinker, I believe that what the liquor world cried out for was a new drink that celebrated the cashmere concept. And here it is, the "Cashmere-tini" —simply ask for the most expensive gin that the bartender or liquor store has available, and have your martini made from that. Just as the occasional cashmere sweater is a necessary indulgence, so too is very expensive, handmade gin. Julia Child may be devoted to her Gordon's gin, but my heart belongs to Hendrick's, recently declared the best of the handmade gins by the *Wall Street Journal*. For a fast giggle on an otherwise dull day in the office, go visit their website at www.cucumbergin.com and you will fall in love with their wit and style, too. Once I developed the complicated formula for the "Cashmere-tini," I realized that I needed a drink for those days when I was out of expensive gin. It hardly ever happens, but a girl needs to be prepared. On those days I'll be drinking a "GinSander" —a gin martini with a lavender sprig floating on top for an aromatic touch. A "GinSander" makes a lovely, lazy summertime pleasure. As if the gin wouldn't relax you enough.

France and was much influenced by many aspects of French life, both at the table and in the bedroom. No doubt it kept him healthy, as he lived to a ripe old age of eighty-three at a time when most did not. That would not have surprised French scientist Selwyn St. Leger, who twenty years ago published a study showing that the French had a much lower heart disease rate than citizens from other countries who consume equally rich food. St. Leger is not alone in his findings, either. There have been many studies both before and since that back up his findings.

Not only does wine have a beneficial effect on our hearts, but it also appears to have a positive effect on that most vexing medical problem—the common cold. According to a Harvard University study, men and women who drank more than fourteen glasses of wine a week caught colds much less often than their nondrinking counterparts, fully 40 percent less!

The Science of Self-Indulgence

Wine labels generally contain the warning "contains sulfites." Sounds scary. Should we be concerned about that? Not at all, says Karen MacNeil, author of The Wine Bible. "Wine has always contained sulfites. . . the compounds occur as a natural by-product of fermentation." Sulfites were once thought to be the cause of wine drinkers' headaches, but current research suggests instead that wine-related headaches have more to do with the individual drinker's difficulty metabolizing it.

Our Friends, the Polyphenols

Yes, just like chocolate, wine contains polyphenols. You remember our friends the polyphenols from just a few pages ago, don't you? Those nice and powerful antioxidants that are the specific nutritional component of wine that provides health benefits. There are other nutritional sources of polyphenols (we've already talked about chocolate), but none comes close to what is found in red wine. Although white wine contains some benefit, it is really red wine that packs a wallop. Red wine has five times the amount of polyphenols that white wine contains. Grapes themselves contain polyphenols, but your basic glass of grape juice doesn't do the trick the same way wine does. The aging process raises the polyphenol bar—the contact between the grape skins and the grape seeds during fermentation concentrates them further. Aging in oak barrels is also thought to increase the levels of polyphenols found in wine.

Of great interest to scientists lately is the idea that red wine contains a substance called resveratrol. Not found in every kind of wine, mind you, resveratrol can occur in high concentrations in wines such as Cabernet Sauvignon and Syrah, and it is thought to be one of the most potent antioxidants yet discovered. Interestingly, it is found in highest concentrations in wines made from grapes grown in cooler climates.

Wine Is Food

In France, wine is considered a food. It is simply a part of the entire meal and meant to be enjoyed as such, not kept separate and special for just the right occasion. Some Americans only drink a glass of wine in a restaurant, or only on the weekends. Can you imagine partaking in a healthy food only on a special occasion? If you don't already, please do incorporate more frequent enjoyment of wine into your meals. When practicing Rule #1—**Eat Only the Very Best**, please make sure you drink the very best alongside it in moderate amounts. Create a newly slim and healthy lifestyle focused on the pleasures of the table, and give a bottle of wine a prime spot at the center of it.

I am such a committed red wine drinker that I formed an eating club around it. Once a month, we members of Red Wine/Black Dresses gather around the hostess's table and raise our glasses high. Not only do we have a wonderful time, but, as I've never once heard a sneeze at the table, it is also clear we all have a much lower incidence of colds!

Recommended Daily Allowance

Even with countless studies that irrefutably prove alcohol is good for you, the chances that your own doctor will ever recommend you drink a glass or two of wine or gin are slim. As you may have noticed, we don't live in France. We are here in the United States of America, which has its wonderful charms as well as its odd quirks. A deep Puritanical streak is one of our nation's quirks. And the Puritanical feelings about "demon liquor" run so deeply that it has at times even colored medical research. The French scientist I quoted in the beginning of this chapter, Selwyn St. Leger, made his discovery about the benefits of wine in the 1980s. American medical researchers had actually discovered it several years before but were asked to keep it quiet.

The Framingham Heart Study began in Framingham, Massachusetts, in 1948. Five thousand residents of that town participated in this ambitious study, which is still underway almost sixty years later. In 1974 a report on factors related to coronary disease was prepared, and the study data showed that there was a strong reduction in the risk of death associated with moderate alcohol consumption. The senior staff at the National Institutes of Health saw this data and asked that it be removed, worried that it would be "socially undesirable in view of the major health problem of alcoholism that already exists in this country."

Not every doctor is quiet on the topic of wine and health. Curtis R. Ellison, M.D., professor of medicine and public health at Boston University School of Medicine, is such a pro-wine person that he has penned articles for magazines such as *Wine Spectator*. Although he doesn't advise women who have a drinking problem to start up again, or women whose religion forbids alcohol to flout the rules, he does feel that "a woman who drinks a glass of wine a day is doing herself a favor. If the practice is sustained, it is beneficial."

Fat Is Just Fine

"Fat gives things flavor," Julia Child says, and as we have vowed to **Eat Only the Very Best** on the Martini Diet, that means we will eat only the most flavorful. Thankfully, fat too has been largely redeemed by scientists of late. We've all learned that lower fat in the diet does not necessarily result in lower fat on the body and that higher fat in our diets doesn't necessarily result in more fat on those same bodies. And, as with chocolate and wine, certain fats are actually beneficial for your heart. The fats found in olive oils and other nut oils, and even in our beloved cheeses, actually assist cancer-fighting agents such as beta-carotene. Working together, fats allow your body to absorb the beta-carotenes you need.

Fat not only gives flavor, helping us abide by Rule #1, it is also vital to satiety. It makes us feel full and gives us the signal to stop eating, so that we can easily abide by Rule #2—**Eat Somewhat Less of the Very Best**.

Holy Guacamole

You may recall that I believed guacamole was my beauty secret in my younger years. No, I didn't put it on my face; like a good California girl, I ate the wonderful stuff. Turns out I wasn't such a silly blonde after all. Avocados have monosaturated fats, and if you are going to eat fat, this is the way to go. Monounsaturated fats give the body signals to make less of the "bad" LDL cholesterol but to leave the "good" HDL cholesterol we all need alone. Nice things really were happening inside my body as I scooped a bit of guac onto a chip. Even nicer, avocados are a tremendous source of vitamin C, vitamin B^6, potassium, and the powerful antioxidant, vitamin E.

Fishing for Compliments

Another fat you hear about in the news on a regular basis is omega-3 fatty acid. This form of fat has huge health benefits in that it lowers blood pressure, thins blood, dilates blood vessels, raises the "good" HDL levels, and fights cancer. Salmon and swordfish are both rich in omega-3, and they are among my favorite dishes (you can find my family's salmon recipe in chapter eight, "My Favorite Indulgences."). Grill salmon for dinner a few times a week and thrive.

As if I haven't gone on about the French enough in this book, I also want to mention the well-known "French Paradox." The paradox being that, although the French typically consume a diet higher in fats than Americans, especially in saturated fats such as dairy products (think cheese and cream), they do not have as high an incidence of heart disease. Could it be that they eat and drink in moderation and do not snack?

The Science of Self-Indulgence

Fat has been studied for centuries. In 1894, the first pronouncements about fat appeared—a USDA scientist recommended that Americans limit their fat intake to 33 percent of their total diet. In 1968, the American Heart Association called for 30 to 35 percent. In 1977, a Senate Select Committee on Nutrition and Human Needs recommended less than 30 percent total fat. In 1997, a Boston-based Nurses Health Study announced that it was not so much total fat as the type of fat consumed. The artificial fats such as the trans fat found in fast foods, crackers, and donuts, are much riskier for your heart than the saturated fats found in butter, cheese, and beef. The American Heart Association announced that year that it would still encourage people to reduce their total fat intake to 30 percent. Julia Child's famous comment that "if you're afraid of butter, as so many people are nowadays, just put in cream!" underscores the very real fear that did develop around butter for a time. Vilified and passed over by many in favor of margarine, butter is now understood to be a natural and balanced fat containing a good dose of monounsaturated fat and few polyunsaturates. Those folks who did switch to margarine for health reasons were wrong—margarine contains trans fat. In 2002, the National Academy of Sciences reported that no amount of trans fat is safe.

Has your brain had enough science for one day? Mine certainly has. Much as I adore wine, chocolate, butter, and cream, and indulge in them regularly, I find I sometimes need indulgences of a different, non-food kind to get me through the ordinariness of daily life. Why don't we move from the science of food and wine to the art of self-indulgence and pampering?

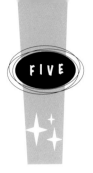

FIVE

Top-shelf Indulgences

Delayed gratification. Now there is an unpleasant term, nearly as unpleasant as "the doctor will see you now," or, "I'm sorry, but we don't have that in your size." Dieters are always piously urged to delay their gratification, to wait for the rewards of a smaller body before they buy new clothes or enjoy their soon-to-be-improved life. Why ever should we delay treating ourselves well and pampering the body we have now? Take matters into your own hands right away and create the indulgent life you dream of.

We've been talking about food and eating for some time now, not unexpected in a diet book, I guess. But aren't you tired of focusing on the idea that you are somehow dissatisfied with the way you look and how delicious life will be once you get it all right? I know I'm tired of writing about it. Instead, let's take a chapter to focus on indulging ourselves in a different way. Indulging our bodies and our minds with new ways of treating ourselves, new ways of behaving, new ways of thinking. Just as a bartender reaches to the top shelf for the Hendrick's gin, for the best liquor he has to offer you, let's stand on our tippy toes and reach up to the high shelf marked "indulgences" and see what we can enjoy right now. All you need is to decide that you do, indeed, deserve it. I know I do, and I know you do, too.

Do your emotions sometimes drive you toward the Krispy Kremes? It's no secret that many of us have boredom, depression, or simmering dissatisfaction at the base of our food pyramid. Think what might happen if those feelings were channeled away from food and toward pampering ourselves. Perhaps serenity, beauty, and luxury might quickly seem an even better option than a glazed donut.

A properly indulgent attitude extends far beyond food, eating, exercise, and weight loss; it is a way of viewing the world and the way we operate in it. Let's start with the way you dress, my dear, and see how easily it can be refocused in a more luxurious way. Come with me to Diva School, training ground of the Martini Way.

In chapter one, I shared the story of how, unhappy at age forty, I reshaped and redirected my life by christening myself "Gin." I also encouraged you to go ahead and buy the beautiful clothes you've denied yourself for years because somehow, someway, you've been led to believe you only deserve to buy top-quality things in small sizes. By now I know you've chosen that sophisticated and adventurous new name for yourself, haven't you? And your eye is drawn to the racks of designer clothes and the shelves of swanky shoes, isn't it? That martini mood will soon give you a huge self-esteem boost as you begin to view yourself in a whole, new, sophisticated way.

The Indulgent Lifestyle

The Martini Diet Rule #1, **Eat Only the Very Best,** is a fine and handy metaphor for how to incorporate the Martini lifestyle into your daily routine. While vowing to henceforth eat only incredible food and avoid the junky things that surround us, it won't be long before your newly developed food snob persona starts to raise its nose at a few other substandard parts of your life.

Living the Martini Lifestyle

 Once you begin to raise the standards you apply to what goes in your mouth, why ever would you want to make the following mistakes: Dress and look just like everyone else in your neighborhood? Drive the same car as everyone else in your neighborhood? Design your pool just like everyone in your neighborhood? And once you apply portion control to how much of the wonderful food you eat, why ever would you: Buy too much of something you don't need? Spend your money on something you can't really afford? The higher your nose goes in the air about food, the higher it will go about everything around you. You are strong enough, brave enough, to be different.

You need to start wearing more cashmere, my dear, to use a phrase I just happened to coin myself some years ago. To remind myself that I needed to take care of myself in the same way I took care of everyone else in my life—my children, my husband, my house, my garden—I posted a little note to myself, "Wear More Cashmere" on my computer, and ever since then I have taken those words to heart. I do indulge myself with the occasional cashmere sweater (because what could be more luxurious than that?), but I also take care to do little things for myself, such as spritz my sheets with lavender sheet spray before climbing in at night, put the perfume strips that come in every magazine into my underwear drawer for a little perfume treat, and join a speaking club so that I can hear regular applause for myself (a most delicious and calorie-free feeling, I assure you).

Why should I have all the fun? I want you to live this way, too. I want you to value who you are now, to hold yourself in high regard and decide that you deserve the very best, and to take immediate steps to incorporate the "cashmere" into your daily life.

Bye Bye Beige

Everyone and everything around us is starting to look pretty humdrum in a beige sort of way, don't you agree? Khaki houses, beige cars, and off-white sweaters; we are all fading quickly into the scenery around us. Why not stand out with a dramatic fashion statement that says—Me? I'm living the Martini lifestyle! What can you wear to feel instantly like someone who has broken out of the beige pack? A big pair of sunglasses, a silk scarf, and elbow-length kidskin leather gloves would certainly do the trick there, don't you think?

Gloves do have such a glamorous and retro feel. Wearing lovely gloves will not only make you feel like a star but will also keep you from snacking, as you don't want to stain the things. Chapter six will give you more ideas on how to avoid overeating and constant snacking, but the glove trick is certainly worth knowing now.

Spidery high heels and big jewelry will also do the trick. Why choose to go through life fading into the background when you can choose to stand out against it? As a young girl, I would shake my head in wonder at older women who were wearing just a bit too much rouge, whose pants were just a shade too bright for their age, and whose jokes were a teensy bit too racy for polite company. But now I realize the very real rewards of being different, of the tawdry thrill of wearing armloads of pearl bracelets with worn jeans and a T-shirt. Sure, the stodgy neighbors may raise their eyebrows at us, but who is having more fun? I say we are. Even when wandering out in public in our mommy costumes of sensible khaki and washable cotton, why not add a touch of sass by slipping into a pair of shoes that will make you feel tall, thin, and a teensy bit naughty? Chances are no one will ever look down and notice.

Hold your breath and go over the top with some really fabulous fashion statement. What have you got to lose? I have a wonderful friend who has been bravely battling cancer for many years. Rather than mope around the house in a robe and slippers, Jane sallies forth in public wearing a pair of red leather jeans and large chunky jewelry she designed herself. She calls them "Janestones" and feels vibrant and strong when she wears them (check them out on www.janestones.com).

Fading into the background is something that, henceforth, you will not do. Stand up, stand straight, stand out, and you will be able to stand the praise and compliments that will soon begin to flow your way.

The Privacy of Your Own Home

If you can't quite summon the nerve to stand out in public yet (and I'm going to continue to encourage you so you'll have to break down eventually), why not indulge in a little fashion fantasy in private?

Another super sexy way to celebrate the body you have now is to wear a sarong around the house. Sarongs are those knotted yards of fabric that Hawaiian and Tahitian women sashay around in. Sure, you could save that swath of fabric and wear it only by the pool, but if it feels so exotic, why not indulge in that feeling while doing the laundry? In a sarong, you walk differently; your hips will sway and swish. It does feel wonderful and reminds you how sexy you are, no matter what your size.

What's that you say? You don't have a sarong? Well, rather than wait until you take an exotic beach vacation and find a cute one in the gift shop, why not make one out of some slinky and sexy fabric? Sarongs for poolside are made out of tropical print cotton, but why not make yourself a fancier version out of lightweight velvet or heavy silk? The dimensions of a full-length sarong are 62 inches by 42 inches and make a big rectangle. Wrap the long side around your waist, grab the two edges up, and tie across your hip. Too sexy.

Get Thee to a Beadery

I love pearls, absolutely love them. But have you ever priced out even a single strand of pearls from a top company such as Mikimoto? Goodness, you could buy a car with that money. I've managed to feed my own pearl addiction much less expensively and at the same time bring a wonderfully indulgent air into my daily routine. My wrists are heavily hung with big chunky pearl bracelets that I made myself, sitting quietly and knotting the silk string at The Bead Shoppe, my local bead store here in Granite Bay. I love the feeling of heavy pearls sliding against my bare skin as I move. It makes even lowly typing feel glamorous and helps keep my hands out of the cookie jar. Come to think of it, these pearl bracelets are so big my hand might not even fit into the cookie jar.

Bead stores aren't just filled with plastic beads for little girls. In addition to freshwater pearls of all sizes and shapes, big girls will find luxurious precious stones such as rubies and sapphires to string, and semiprecious stones including amethyst and garnets to knot together into luscious strands. The more glamorous you feel, the less likely you are to overindulge in weak moments. You look like a star, you act like a star, and soon, you will have the body of a star.

Side by Side

Now that you are becoming more indulgent in your own approach to life and dress and food, can you share this with the man in your life? Heavens, I would hope so! It may take you a while to bring him around to your new food rules, so why not begin by getting him involved in your new indulgent exercise routines? Riding, skating, and fencing may well have been things he dreamed about too in his younger years, and including him would give him a chance to recapture a bit of romance and adventure in his life, too. While you are posting along in a velvet helmet and tight-fitting hacking jacket, imagining you resemble the young Jackie Kennedy, your man can embrace his chance to sit astride a big snorting beast and imagine himself as the Lord of the Manor. We aren't the only ones with a vivid fantasy life, you know...

"Exercise is lonely, working on yourself by yourself. Dancing isn't a lonely pursuit at all!" says Barbara Nicholas, a ballroom dance instructor. She and her husband teach many couples the basics of ballroom dancing. Barbara points out that compared to working out together in a gym there is a real advantage to the dance floor: "The men are better dressed, and they smell better, too!" Another advantage that may well help you convince your partner to join you is that "dancing can be extremely romantic; it's kind of like foreplay."

The Science of Self-Indulgence

Regular exercise helps you relax—you already know that. Regular exercise with your lover (maybe you can get him to take up fencing, too; he might look good in one of those puffy shirts) may be even more relaxing, though. A study at The Monell Chemical Senses Center in Philadelphia discovered that men's armpit sweat calms women. Volunteers reported feeling less tense and more relaxed as they sniffed.

Clean and Shiny

As indulgent as working out in tandem can be (particularly if it is on a polished wooden ballroom floor), imagine this equally indulgent scenario—dusting off your jodhpurs, you return from a riding lesson and open the front door to your home and breathe deeply. Ah, the smell of lemon furniture polish wafts out. It seems that while you were out, the cleaning lady was in.

Mmmm, heaven here on earth. Yes, of course it is expensive and frivolous, but do try to arrange it at least once as a treat. Even if you do your own cleaning (and girls, I mostly do mine), as a special indulgence arrange to have someone come in while you are out working on yourself.

If the only furniture polish you ever get to smell is what you've rubbed on the end tables yourself, a less opulent (but equally indulgent) way to perfume the air is with the many candles that have food-related scents. I find that the smell of a caramel scented candle (yes, I really have one) keeps me from feeling deprived when I'm avoiding dessert. Your house will smell like a dinner party has just ended and your happy guests have gone home with a taste of blueberry tart on their lips. Scented candles seem to be sold everywhere nowadays. My local grocery store really does sell a blueberry tart-scented candle, as well as apple turnover and praline cream. Such a luscious smell in the house.

Close your eyes and imagine the luxury of a calm, quiet, clean, and lightly scented home. Take a deep breath and picture the new life you are building for yourself. In this serene and elegant setting, why ever would you sully it with a bag of Doritos? There would simply be no need to sedate your emotions with fatty snacks.

Give Yourself an Upgrade

No doubt there are many committed fingernail fanciers among you, but I've long felt that weekly manicures are more than a little pointless. An hour spent in a crowded shop breathing in all those ghastly chemicals, only to have your polish chip the next day. Why not try this instead for a few months: Buy a $2 bottle of nail polish in a neutral color and do your own nails for a few months, and then take the few hundred dollars you'll save and put it to use for a bigger, more luxurious purpose.

First off, I suggest you upgrade both your sheets and your underwear.

Slipping in between high-thread-count cotton sheets at night is a tremendous reward for abiding by those restrained and refined Martini Diet rules, isn't it? The only thing better might be sleeping in what Marilyn Monroe once happily announced she wore to bed—nothing but Chanel No. 5. Price out high-thread-count sheets at your local bedding store and you just might reach for a Krispy Kreme to revive yourself. Top-quality sheets are not that expensive when you seek them out on sale, though, or at closeout warehouses. A wonderful place to find them is at the national bargain chain, Tuesday Morning. That store seems to have an entire aisle devoted to expensive sheets delightfully discounted; a set of Egyptian cotton sheets with a silky 500 thread count is only $159. See how easy it is? Skip ten manicures and sleep like a princess!

Underneath It All

Top-quality lingerie will make you always aware that, underneath your clothes, you are indulging in great style. A fine and secret pleasure, indeed. Fond as I am of buying designer clothes for less at consignment stores or online through eBay, I realize that lingerie is vastly different from a Chanel suit worn once or twice by someone else. Go straight to the lingerie section in your favorite top-dollar department store and spend away. Celebrate your body by covering it in satin, silk, and lace. The wonderful thing about this indulgence is that even very expensive lingerie is within reach of most budgets. All it takes is the permission to yourself to indulge in a way that is sweetly secret for many hours of the day. Because what kind of a message are you sending yourself by wearing that tatty old underwear everyday, anyway? Tell yourself how very much you are worth, right now, as you are. Send your self-esteem a valentine with silk and lace.

What else can you upgrade in your life? You are going to **Eat Only the Very Best** from now on, so perhaps you should apply that to other areas of your life as well. Start off by choosing a smallish area in your life, not cars or audio equipment, which will cost many thousands to upgrade. Instead upgrade the brand of coffee or tea you drink every morning.

Upgrade the way you view what you deserve out of life, and the luscious goodies hidden up on the top shelf of life will soon be yours.

A Quiet Hush

Our daily lives are so riddled with rude interruptions, from the distant sound of a car horn to the chirp of the cell phone ringing next to you in a darkened movie theater. When living the Martini lifestyle, I hope you'll join me in turning your back on all this nonsense. You have an incredible meal to enjoy, so unplug the phone. You have a lover who needs your attention, so turn off the television. You have a life to enjoy, so sign off your computer. Make sure that there are large parts of your day devoted to simple enjoyment of food, friends, and family, without the distraction of the outside world. Indulge them all with your attention.

Living the Martini Lifestyle

 In a grocery store aisle not long ago I stumbled upon a way to feel instantly younger! Sound impossible? Not if you buy your cosmetics at the teen counter. All of those flavored, scented Chapsticks make me feel like I'm in junior high school and I'm hoping that cute blond boy Greg will kiss me after school. The smell of cherry, strawberry, or vanilla takes me straight back to the age of fourteen. Wait, I'm even close to remembering the combination of my locker!

Indulgent Beauty

With all this indulgence gently lapping into your new life like the soft waves on a Hawaiian beach, where else can you improve? Your life is on its way to being indulgent; can you indulge your looks as well? Swank (yet affordable) beauty treatments abound for you to enjoy. Indulge away, my dears.

Rubs You the Right Way

You didn't need to buy a copy of *The Martini Diet* to know that spas and massages are deliciously indulgent ways to pamper yourself. But do you really give yourself permission to go there, to actually indulge in a facial, a body scrub, or a massage? Be honest now. Spas are lavish and expensive places to spend your time and money, and a trip to the spa is the very sort of thing that we dangle in front of ourselves in order to force ourselves to accomplish something. *No, no, I can't have a massage unless I lose five pounds first. No, no, I can't have a facial until I can run three miles without stopping.* Oh, please. Put this book down now and book yourself a facial. A mini-facial, anyway, if you can't quite get the pleasure thing going yet.

Although I have the pleasure thing going in a major way, I confess that I've never been on one of those indulgent week-long spa vacations where the whole point is to be pampered and primped. A spa morning, of course, a spa afternoon, indeed, even an evening in a spa (with my husband, Peter, on the outdoor massage table next to mine) all leading up to a whole weeks' worth of attention someday. You don't have to wait for me to get there first, though. I'm encouraging you to surge past me in this indulgence category, to sprint ahead (which wouldn't be hard, considering the thin and spindly high heels I mince around in) and book yourself for a week of pleasure. Send me a postcard.

Sound too lavish for words? Need I remind you that this is something you deserve, regardless of where you are now in life. Permission to pamper is hereby granted.

A Ritzy Afternoon

The name "Ritz-Carlton" is an internationally known symbol for luxury. And it sounds like a place that most of us can't really afford. Well, if you aren't up to the room rate at the Ritz or the swanky hotel nearest your house, why not just visit their day spa? A room may run into the several hundreds, but you can be pampered and indulged by the same spa staff as their overnight guests for far less than that.

The Ritz-Carlton at Half Moon Bay in Northern California is set dramatically at the edge of a windswept cliff above the pounding surf, but all is cool and calm in the confines of their gracious day spa. I spent a relaxing afternoon there not long ago in a diligent effort to investigate the latest in spa services. As I am encouraging you to go forth and indulge yourself in life, I thought it only right that I should rather selflessly undergo the rigors first before suggesting that you do.

Is there a better way to spend two hours and $200? I can't imagine one right offhand. Padding around in a sumptuous spa robe and slippers, taking advantage of the whirlpool and sauna while waiting for my appointment? Heaven. It was really just the price of a new pair of shoes. Shoe diva that I am, even I can see the wisdom in occasionally choosing instead to spend the money lying quietly on a padded massage table while a well-trained person pampers me shamelessly.

The kind and generous Spa at the Ritz-Carlton at Half Moon Bay would like to share a recipe similar to the popular treatment their spa is known for.

Pumpkin Body Mask

2 Tbsp oatmeal
½ cup (120ml) heavy cream
¼ cup (60g) canned or fresh pumpkin
2 Tbsp cornmeal
2 Tbsp honey

In a mixing bowl, grind the oats. Add the remaining ingredients and mix to form a paste. Apply the mask from the neck down (including the arms, legs, tummy, and glutes), using light strokes. Wrap your body in a cotton sheet and wait ten minutes lying down (the mask will not stain). Rinse off the mask in a warm bath or shower. Pat dry and apply a moisturizer to nourish. The result? Healthy and glowing skin!

Same Old, Same Old

I grew up in the stodgy world of old California money. Old money is not like new money, which gets spent on face-lifts and first class tickets. Old money doesn't actually get spent, you see, which is how it gets to be so old. And the women in my world, in addition to not spending money on face-lifts and first class, chose a plain and sensible hairstyle in the seventh grade and then stuck with it for the next seventy years. And so I stuck with long blonde hair without much style until I was in my mid-thirties. It was a cheeky hairdresser who, when I asked for a basic trim, sighed loudly and said, "Couldn't we do something just a little more modern?" My haughty hackles up, I took the bait and an hour later emerged a new woman. What the heck had been holding me back? A new hairstyle (or brave, new color) can instantly make you feel like a new person with a new body and a new outlook (a Martini outlook) on life.

A Brand New You

Have you ever walked by the makeup section of a large department store during a cosmetics company promotion and seen the make up artists standing by, waiting to brush your cheeks with the latest in radiant blush? Girls, those makeup artists aren't there waiting for someone else to sit down in the model's chair—they are waiting for you! Don't be one of those shy shoppers, loitering around on the edges of the demonstration, waiting until someone catches your eye, hoping to be invited over to participate.

Invite yourself. Go up and ask for what you want and need out of life, my dear. Whether it is a free makeup job or a promotion, don't wait for someone to ask you!

Relax and let the makeup artist do what she will with your face. You can pretend for twenty minutes that you are a model being readied for a big shoot. You may not like the result, the colors may not be what you are used to, but it is a lovely way to bust out of the same old makeup routine you've been putting on your face for years. I just confessed that I wore the same dull hairstyle for decades, and I still have the same eye makeup kit I bought in college. I need to be busted out of my beauty routine with regularity, and I'm guessing you could benefit, too. How do you find out when these free makeup sessions arise? Ask the makeup counter staff to put you on the mailing list for events.

Hot Sundae Nights

Did all of that chocolate talk a few chapters back whet your appetite for the dark dreaminess of a mug of hot chocolate? What if I told you it was possible to have a full-body hot chocolate experience? The perfect scented bath for a lazy Sunday is a tub of hot chocolate to soak in, and it is made like this:

Mix together 2 Tbsp of an inexpensive brand of unsweetened cocoa powder, ½ cup of dry milk powder, and ½ cup of unscented bubble bath. Toss the ingredients under the tap of a hot running bath and mix the water vigorously to make it frothy and lump-free. Slip in and relax.

Living the Martini Lifestyle

 The Spa at the Ritz-Carlton in Half Moon Bay, California, isn't the only one working with the powerful pumpkin. Jeanne Marie, the founder of International Media Cosmetics, has worked with the top faces in media and politics, from Diane Sawyer and Peter Jennings to Bill Clinton and Al Gore, getting them ready for their television close-ups.

"And who really likes the way they look in a close shot anyway?" Jeanne Marie laughs. "Makeup can only do so much. My clients also wanted a product that would help them look visibly younger. I developed the Pumpkin Peel to help. Pumpkin not only tastes yummy, but it also has all kinds of things in it that are good for your skin when applied topically—it contains the highest form of beta-carotene around." Check out Jeanne's website at www.pumpkinpeel.com to order dessert for your face.

I can see you now, slathered with pumpkin, your hips swathed in a sexy sarong you found at the back of your closet, wrists heavy with pearls and sapphires, and the room heavy with the scent of sweet apple candles. Food? We haven't thought about it for the last hour. Who needs it, when there is lavish jewelry to be worn? Who needs the false comfort of a late-night bowl of ice cream when your self-esteem is as high as your elegantly spiky shoes? But this is a diet book after all, girls; it is time to totter in our high heels back over to the main topic of losing weight in an indulgent way.

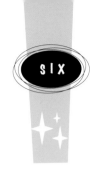

SIX

Cinnabon Avoidance Techniques

Ooooo, that smell is absolutely irresistible. It takes all my inner strength to ignore it whenever it appears in the air. Yes, you know the smell I mean—that sweet, yeasty, caramel, and cinnamon odor that trails across the airport terminal in your direction, seducing you to abandon your carefully packed matched set of luggage at the gate just before boarding and rush with your arms and your wallet wide open towards those cinnamon rolls dripping with freshly made glaze.

Time and time again I have politely pointed out in these pages that snacking leads us down a chunky path and must be eliminated from our daily eating habits. As much as I am urging you to adopt a refined, elegant, restrained attitude toward food, and though snacking is by no means refined, elegant, or restrained, there *are* times when to err truly is human. How to avoid erring, then, human as we girls are?

I'd like to share with you some of the Cinnabon avoidance techniques I've developed for myself over the years. Cinnabon avoidance? I know I'm not the only one out there who trembles inside at the smell of a warm cinnamon bun dripping with gooey cream (and I have been known to ask for extra topping!). Even in my most stringent noncarb dieting phase I was weakened and powerless in their presence. And what is your secret snacking weakness? I know you have one. It might also be cinnamon rolls fresh out of the oven, or perhaps it is the basket of chips in a Mexican restaurant, a package of a dozen fat-free cookies, or the sugar-glazed calling card of the diet devil—Krispy Kremes. Oh, I could go on and on about the many temptations that surround us in this snack-food world, but I fear it might send you to your cupboard, so I will cease it at once. Instead, let's focus on how to turn away from the tempting and keep our minds more firmly where they belong—on living the Martini Diet lifestyle.

Such Minty-fresh Breath You Have!

For the weak-willed, a powerful way to beat the snacking demons is always to carry around those tiny breath strips that melt on your tongue. The moment you sniff cinnamon rolls or fudge brownies, pull one out and pop it in. The tiny strong mints will do as well. The point is to blast your mouth with mint and you simply won't want to eat after that. It really wouldn't taste very good.

The same technique works well if you are trying (and failing) to scale back the amount you are eating during meals. When you reach the point in your meal when you think you should stop (but lack the discipline), just do the mint thing. Although many a lavish dinner is broken up between courses by a palate cleanser that leaves you looking forward to the next course (the French call it an *amuse bouche*, which means "amuse the mouth"), these breath strips work as palate killers instead. Eeeech! You will lose your desire to pick up your fork and dive back in after one of those. Try not to let your hostess see you doing this—please be subtle. But at home you can do it whenever you need to, without worrying about hurting anyone's feelings.

The Pie Pixies

One of my own weaknesses in life (please don't be fooled by my couture-wearing schoolmarm tone in this book, I am full of failings and weaknesses) is dessert. If I order coffee after dinner there is a very good chance I will succumb to the dessert demons. My brain thinks, "First a sip of coffee, then a bite of something sweet."

I've already confessed my deep and abiding love of pie (a serious weakness indeed when it comes to wearing a small size). I love pie, just love it. That after-dinner cup of coffee, it just cries out for a side of pie with a scoop of ice cream balanced on top. Not something in which I can indulge daily, is it? Rather than skip my coffee entirely I have found a seasonally acceptable way to keep pie at a distance: iced coffee. Ordering black iced coffee after dinner lets me get my coffee fix, and somehow an iced drink doesn't make me crave a crumbly cobbler or a peachy pie.

If you are also a coffee-and-sweet girl, try this method. If it doesn't work, I'm afraid you may have to skip that after-dinner coffee entirely.

Pay for Removal

Some years ago, I was enjoying a pleasant lunch at a Northern California steak joint with Van Gordon Sauter, bon vivant and retired media mogul (he's the former president of CBS News and was the bureau chief of the Paris news division for many years in the sixties). Van likes to eat—I don't think he'd mind my telling you that. His approach to eating dessert, though, is unique. When placing his order (I have total recall when it comes to desserts; it was a fudge brownie topped with three types of Häagen Dazs ice cream), he turned his stern gaze upon the young waitress and said, "Now dear, you need to understand that the size of your tip today while depend on how quickly you snatch this away from me after I begin eating." Needless to say, she was more than a little startled by his request, but gamely took it to heart by whisking the dessert plate away from him after he'd taken six or seven bites. "Perfect!" he declared, and did leave a large tip indeed. So, for those of us who lack the will power to skip dessert entirely, we can always pay the waiter to set our limits for us.

Keep Your Hands on the Wheel, Please

I've touched on this before—you *really* need to give up eating and drinking in the car. It isn't elegant, it isn't adult, it isn't at all refined. Not only will you skip those extra calories once you give up eating in the car, but you also won't risk muffin crumbs on the carpet and chocolate smudges on your blouse. Difficult as it is, you should also try to wean your children from the habit.

Why am I so rigid about this? Because you are trying to adopt a whole new attitude toward food. That food is something to indulge in and enjoy every time you approach it, not just something to rush through and catch between appointments. To resist the urge to partake on the run, remember to focus on those mental images of thin and stylish women. WWJD? What Would Jackie Do? She would certainly not have eaten an Egg 95 in the front seat of her car while driving between appointments at the doctor and the hairdresser. Or try to imagine any other stylish, thin woman—say, Katharine Hepburn—munching on a bag of chips as she waited for a light to change. This no eating in the car rule extends to drinking coffee, water, and soda, too. And then, after you have eliminated this habit from your life, you just might feel the need to indulge and reward yourself with a better car to fit your new life!

Bright White Smile

Here is a marvelous way not only to avoid snacking but also to make a real change in your appearance at the same time. Whiten your teeth with those little strips! Do your moments of weakness always happen at the same time of day? Why not decide to put those little strips on at around the same time and foil your cravings? Wearing the strips actually prevents you from eating and drinking for up to an hour at a time (you wear each strip for thirty minutes, and you can do a second set for another thirty minutes right away if you want). Your teeth feel so nice and clean afterward that you just may not want to eat right away. If the hours after dinner are when you are most likely to break down and eat a carton of French vanilla ice cream, whiten instead. If mid-morning is when you most struggle with the desire to snack between meals, do it then. After the two weeks it takes to go through a box of whitening strips, you'll not only have a brighter smile but also better cheekbones to go with it!

Choose One

If you are a lifelong snacker you may not be able to forgo it all at once. The cold-turkey approach may be too difficult, particularly if a slice of cold turkey left over from dinner is what beckons to you later in the night. So go ahead and ease into it by giving up some things, but not others. Perhaps the first few weeks you could vow to give up your morning munch of a donut or two. Once you get used to that you could move on to the later parts of the day and clean up the snacking habit hour by hour. Since we are indulgent women, choose one thing that you won't give up at all, but will allow yourself to indulge in on occasion. You might give up the early evening cheese and crackers but allow yourself a spoonful of ice cream as a treat later on. As a rigid and disciplined young woman, I gave up potato chips, soda, and French fries from the time I turned thirteen until I was in college in an effort to avoid blemishes (it seemed to work, only to

break out in my thirties!), but I
still allowed myself to snack on
chocolate chip cookies whenever
they turned up.

Be Good in the Morning

I find that if I start the day off well,
with a brisk walk, my fifty standard
situps, and a modest breakfast, I do pretty
well throughout the day. That feeling of pride and accomplishment goes a long way toward helping me toe the line for the rest of the day. But if I start the day off by skipping any exercise and digging into a plate of French toast smothered with butter and maple syrup, there is a good chance the rest of the day will be equally caloric and slothful. Do try to get off to a good start in the morning so that your day goes well, too. Make every effort to get in an early morning workout. Reign in your impulses and sit down to a good breakfast and not only will your day unfold splendidly but your pants will fit, too.

Create an Elegant Atmosphere

When I urge you to skip the junk food and treat yourself to eating only incredible food in modest helpings, I am also picturing you sitting down to a lovely table set with good china and a vase of fresh flowers. If you put the same care and attention into the way your meal is presented, you will never feel deprived, regardless of how modest the serving of crisply baked chicken and freshly picked spinach. Remember that the Martini Diet philosophy is to savor and enjoy your food, not rush through a meal in order to get on with the rest of your day. Indulging in a pleasant meal *is* the rest of your day, so don't rush through it at all. Instead, take the time to set a beautiful table, to put out a pretty china tea mug and matching breakfast bowl, to use lovely worn silver teaspoons you found at a garage sale to add to the atmosphere of refined elegance at your breakfast table.

Even a lunch at your desk can be made into an event you look forward to if you build in rituals of beauty. Perhaps you can buy just one place setting of exceptionally fine china to store at the office and use there at your desk every day to improve the way your lunch hour feels. So often we are overeating to compensate for a feeling of lack, but who would ever feel lacking when seated at a lovely table?

The Science of Self-Indulgence

Breakfast is an important meal for Martini Diet enthusiasts, and research shows that skipping breakfast leads to overeating later in the day. But not every breakfast is good for you. McDonald's new breakfast offering, the McGriddle, weighs in at 550 calories, 33 grams of fat, and 260 milligrams of cholesterol. It also seems to be a big hit with their customers. But you would never eat one, would you? You are far too much of a food snob now, far too good for that sort of thing.

The Hired Help

A recent study showed that, regardless of the actual goal you set out to achieve—monetary, physical, or career—if you hire a personal coach to keep you on track, your chances of success double. Hiring a personal coach to get you through a weight-loss campaign is expensive, of course, but if you have had real trouble in the past changing your habits it may well be just what you need. Why would having a coach make such a difference in the outcome? Personally, I think it is because we hate to disappoint people. Once you and your coach agree that your goal for the week is to lose two pounds, you will do everything in your power to avoid showing up on the appointed day with less than that very result. I'm a people-pleaser, and I bet you are, too. The constant encouragement is worth paying for as well; the friendly (but firm) voice on the phone inquiring after your mid-week progress helps you stay on track. Short of hiring a professional, is there someone in your life who can play this role for you? I recommend looking outside of your own household for a weight-loss coach; regardless of how kind and loving your mate is, you will ultimately resent his questions and attention to what you are eating and when.

The Overindulgence Cure

I went through a phase in my early twenties when I was mad for the white chocolate strawberry truffles at a handmade candy shop that was conveniently around the corner from a bookshop I worked in. I would stand behind the bookshop counter every day, counting the minutes until I could slip over to the shop for yet another piece of that candy. Day after day I ate a truffle or two, and my jeans grew tighter and tighter. What to do? I just couldn't resist them. This habit needed to stop, but how? One day, instead of buying one truffle, I bought six. The first truffle was magnificent. The second one felt like sinful indulgence. The third one gave me a stomachache. The fourth one made me feel dizzy. The fifth and the sixth? Well, let's just say that after I forced myself to eat all six of those white chocolate strawberry truffles I had lost my taste for them. I've used this method a few times since them to break myself of a longing for something; just eat it until it makes you sick. Go ahead and try it on something that you can't resist, something that makes you fall off the modest portion wagon every time you see it. Next time don't even try to resist the siren call. Order it all and sit down and eat until you never want to see that food again.

Go Ahead and Munch

Snacking while cooking is a huge temptation. A little taste of this, a little taste of that, and pretty soon you've had an entire meal before you even sit down to join your family! How can you keep the spoon out of your mouth while working in the kitchen? This is why gum exists. Chewing gum, however inelegant it may be, is a wonderful way to avoid tasting what you are cooking. How's that? Could it be because your mouth is already full, your jaw is already working, and you already have some flavor in your favor, so why would the spaghetti sauce beckon? And if you aren't tasting the food, it gives you a lovely reason to invite your love into the kitchen to have a little taste for you.

Living the Martini Lifestyle

Would you eat any less if you knew that all your friends would soon be seeing much more of you? As in, all of you. One artistic way not only to celebrate the body you have now but also affirm your commitment to living lighter is to have an artist do your portrait. Brave girls (and I know you are a brave girl, aren't you?) will go ahead and pose nude for the artist, and then proudly hang the result in the hallway. Art schools need models, as do working artists, so don't be afraid to suggest yourself.

Don't Stay Still

Doesn't it seem like really thin people just can't sit still? It could be that is why they are so thin. So often "thin and nervous" go together, like those whippet-thin greyhounds who can't even settle their bottoms on the ground. In fact, even the tiniest movements can burn calories. Fidgeting in your seat, tapping your toes under the conference table during a boring meeting, dancing around your living room to a secret song only you can hear, any kind of movement can help you burn up to 100 extra calories a day. Do arm strengthening pushes on your steering wheel while stuck in traffic, clench your butt together at the stoplight, and of course you are doing Kegels in your car, aren't you? Wherever you are, whatever you are doing, add a bit of extra movement and it will all add up to more calories burned throughout the course of an ordinary day. And that, as we know, is a good thing.

A Fine Mist

Here is another fine way to interrupt those thoughts of snacking and derail the desire to eat. Spritz your face with an herbal atomizer. I'm fond of the Burt's Bees Lavender Complexion Mist. It sits in my desk drawer, and in moments of weakness I reach in, close my eyes, and spritz my face with that lovely soft scent. Lavender is a calming herb, of course, so if it is stress and tension that are behind your sudden desire to snack, spending a few peaceful moments inhaling the lavender scent will help immediately. This sounds nutty, but it really does work! You will refresh and hydrate your skin, and the lavender perfume lingers behind to kill your interest in food. The smell of flowers will send your thoughts in a new direction, away from the kitchen and out into an open meadow. There are many facial mists on the market; you might find one with your favorite scent, too.

The Science of Self-Indulgence

Imagine how your life will change once you make a permanent change in your eating habits and watch the weight slowly melt away for good. Slimmer people have an increased life span and a decreased risk of cancer, cardiovascular disease, and diabetes, according to the *International Journal of Toxicology*.

Have a Seat

Another common part of our rush-rush, hurry-hurry life nowadays is the stand-up meal. Along with my belief that you should eat only the very best is my insistence that you

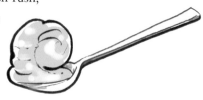

need to be sitting down when you eat it. Honor your food and yourself and take the time to enjoy what you are putting in your mouth; don't stand in the corner of a café wolfing down a bit of muffin.

Vow never again to stand and eat. What would this do to your ability to eat at cocktail parties? It would certainly curtail overeating, wouldn't it, if you decided that from now on you won't stand there with a glass of wine in one hand and a napkin filled with tiny meatballs in the other. Yes, you may eat a thing or two at a cocktail buffet, but take the time to choose a few little appetizers, put them on a plate, find a seat, and focus on the fact that you are eating. Eating while standing up is inattentive eating, something that Martini Diet devotees simply do not do.

The Science of Self-Indulgence

We snack because it feels good, but there is a very real downside. A study appearing in September 2003 in the *Proceedings of the National Academy of Sciences* found that indulging every so often in a cookie to combat stress is fine, but that habitually using comfort foods to combat stress is likely to be bad for your long-term health.

Slinky and Sexy

I've always found that, in order to better appreciate my body and focus on why I want to remain slim, wearing fabrics that let me feel my body when I move is a wonderful touch. Soft and slinky fabrics such as silk, cashmere, and velvet, which drape across my skin and feel so good to the touch make me feel sexy and aware of myself. We can't always wear blue jeans and T-shirts, and floating through life in a drapey dress that makes you feel elegantly alive will help you exercise restraint at the table. You might feel so gorgeous that you will skip the meal entirely. Surround yourself with sensuous fabrics and designs and you will create a whole new persona for yourself. Try out that new name you chose a few chapters back. It might not be Cathleen who wears a black velvet skirt—maybe it is your sexy and adventurous new counterpart, "Cat."

The Science of Self-Indulgence

Apple growers in Washington state, working hand in hand with nutritionists and a Gold's Gym in the apple-growing town of Wenatchee, have developed the three-a-day apple plan. Eat one medium-size apple a half hour before each meal, breakfast, lunch, and dinner, and the fiber in the apple will keep you from overeating during your meal. The participants in the Wenatchee trial lost an average of seventeen pounds in three months. Who doesn't like apples?

A Puff of Sugar

If you just can't do without dessert after a meal and miss that sweet taste in your mouth, then here is something small you can have and still feel satisfied—marshmallows. I'm afraid that the whole S'mores thing (graham crackers, slice of chocolate, and toasted marshmallow) is not acceptable as a nightly event, but at just 50 calories for two, marshmallows by themselves are a lovely little indulgence. Make sure you have the discipline to stop at just two, though. A bag of marshmallows is not a part of the Martini Diet, my dears.

Doggie Style

You've seen all the grim statistics about the size of restaurant meals, about how they have crept up to monstrous proportions in the last few decades. So how do you avoid eating too much in a restaurant? Why not ask for a doggie bag the minute the waiter sets your plate down in front of you? You can make this one huge meal into two smaller meals from the get-go and not have to rely on your willpower if it is cut up and bagged right away. And it is one less meal you will have to prepare. Your lunch or dinner is ready to go for tomorrow.

A Formal Affair

As you may have begun to suspect, I have a deep and abiding interest in clothes. Fancy clothes, couture clothes, clothes that make me feel like a princess, if only for the amount of time I have them on. So what do clothes have to do with food and eating? To ratchet up the glamour of your evening meal and make it a special occasion, why not change into an evening gown or other dressy outfit at night? It will put you in a different mood entirely and let you focus on what is on your plate and how much of it you are eating. If you think your family and friends will tease you about coming to the table in your finery, perhaps you can wait until they are safely in bed and then change. Wearing a glamorous outfit in the evening on an otherwise ordinary night will help you avoid the munching syndrome. Who would sit and eat greasy or gloppy snacks while draped in a favorite dress? Trust me, it works.

The Slow Rub

Another way to occupy yourself during the late-night munching hours is to give a massage. Your partner will be delighted at the attention and, I hope, will return the favor. Like wearing a wonderful dress to avoid eating, covering your hands with scented massage oil will also vastly reduce the chances that you will use those same hands to dip into a bag of salty snacks.

Busy, Busy Hands

I am a nighttime reader, alas, and reading can sometimes lend itself to mindless snacking. It can also lend itself to more glasses of wine than a restrained person should really drink. Instead of nighttime reading, then, I took up needlepoint. Any type of craft that keeps your hands busy—needlepoint, quilting, knitting—helps keep munching at bay. In my own family, my very refined and restrained Auntie Bee sits in her Carmel, California, home knitting peacefully instead of visiting that town's famous restaurants, and her daughter, Mary, knits on the other coast in Princeton, New Jersey. I submit that the sweaters they knit for themselves are smaller sizes because of their crafting habit. My own thin mother needlepointed through the sixties and seventies before taking up quilting in the eighties, and I have never seen her eat between meals. By taking up a craft that requires you to keep your clean, grease-free hands busy, you will also begin to fill up your life with completed art projects, pillows, sweaters, and quilts that you've made yourself. A much better way to spend the evenings than finishing up the leftover lasagna from dinner a few hours before.

Eating in the Air

Remember Barbara Curtis? The Slow Food devotee who would turn up her nose at the junk food that was available during business trips? Like Barbara, I try to avoid most of what is available in airports and hotels. My routine with airline flights is to call a few days before the flight and request a fruit plate instead of the ordinary stuff they serve from the food cart. When flying cross-country, I treat it as an in-flight spa day. Just fruit and plenty of water, then early to bed when I land, and the next day I am feeling sharp (not to mention lighter!).

Go Climb a Rock

When the junk food mood strikes unexpectedly, why not avoid the impulse to snack and instead go outside for a quick bit of fresh air? Rather than joining in the mid-morning donut break at the office, take a quick walk around the parking lot to get your blood pumping and get you out of the same room as the dastardly donuts. Hike up a hill, skip down the street—do anything to move your body instead of your mouth.

Just a Tiny Taste

A wonderful way to sidestep the size of most restaurant meals is to order only from the appetizer menu. Ordering an appetizer and a bowl of soup or a salad will give you a wonderfully varied taste of good food, instead of a huge portion of something that will weigh you down. It not only saves calories; chances are you will save money ordering that way as well.

The Science of Self-Indulgence

Money magazine reported that when three Harvard economists applied economic theory to the question of why Americans are getting so big, they were surprised by what they found. Despite the conventional belief that we are getting fatter because of bigger portions and fattening fast food, the authors maintain it is because of the amount of food we eat due to snacking.

Cinnabon Avoidance Technique

I really do have a way to avoid weighing myself down (literally) with one of those tempting cinnamon rolls at the mall or the airport. If I absolutely can't resist a taste, I order just a tiny cup of extra frosting and eat it with a spoon! That way I've avoided the hundreds of calories that an entire roll contains, and I've satisfied my sweet tooth at the Cinnabon counter with just a hundred or so calories. Try it, along with all the suggestions I've laid out above. Once you get out of the habit of snacking and eating large portions it will all become second nature. You will have embraced the Martini Diet rules and incorporated them into your life. From now on (henceforth, my dears), you will pass gracefully through life with a newly slimmed-down body and a newly superior outlook on life. Enjoy!

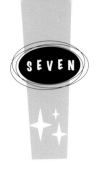

SEVEN

Embrace Indulgence For Life

At last, all the elements of the Martini Diet are firmly in place. Don't knock them over as you reach for your martini glass again, darling. I have carefully constructed these chapters, and I'll thank you not to scatter them all over the floor now. All that hard work investigating the world of indulgent exercise, all those hours carefully concocting the "Cashmere-tini" and the "GinSander", all that berry pie I dutifully pushed away, I'd hate to think that was valuable time wasted.

Similar to the final week at a posh finishing school, let's carefully review all that we have covered in *The Martini Diet: The Self-Indulgent Way to a Thinner, More Fabulous You!* Like all finishing school grads, you are now a committed snob. Not snobbish toward others, I hope and pray, but snobbish toward the dross that surrounds us at the table so often nowadays. The enormous portions of tacky foods riddled with ghastly additives and chemicals and all manner of unhealthy ingredients. The silly foods that are advertised on television and in magazines, sprayed with glycerin to look mouth-watering. The foolish behavior of those who wander around in public, snacking and drinking like small children, unable to control their impulses. You are far, far above such base pursuits.

Our three basic rules of The Martini Diet are:

1. **Eat Only the Very Best**
2. **Eat Somewhat Less of the Very Best**
3. **Eat the Very Best Only at Mealtimes**

Graduates of Martini Manor, our particular posh finishing school, are wholeheartedly committed to eating the very best and most delicious food available, and never darkening the doorway of a fast-food establishment again. When sitting at the table surveying the luscious spread before us, we take modest portions and helpings of the very best, and we eat only until we are satisfied, never stuffed. We only eat three times a day, at the appointed mealtimes; we do not let our hands wander anywhere near the cookie jar on an otherwise dull afternoon.

As for moving our bodies, we do it often and with great relish, because we indulge in forms of exercise that feed our imaginations and our sense of elegance and majesty. We all know that in order to eat extraordinary food we must also commit to making exercise a regular part of our daily lives.

The words elegance, sophistication, refinement, and restraint are hand-stitched into the school emblem of Martini Manor (the school's fancy Latin motto translates to—*Is this my drink?*). I'm so pleased to have you in the graduating class. By reducing portion size, exercising in an indulgent manner, and turning up your nose at the very common and tacky habit of snacking between meals, slowly and carefully the weight will slip off. Which, let us not forget, is indeed our goal. To shed those dumpy pounds that stand between us and a sleek martini glass-like figure. Before we return to the topic of losing weight, though, let's once again visit women's body images.

As you may have begun to suspect, I'm a bit of a fuzzy-sweater feminist. Having started out in my younger years working as a junior lobbyist for a women's organization (even then I stalked the halls of the Capitol building in perilously high heels, draped in silk, with only the most demure of single strand pearls, though, not the over-the-top 12-foot strand I sport now) before wandering over to the business of books, I still harbor many of those same beliefs.

I still firmly believe that you and I are in charge of our own destinies, responsible for our own lives, and perfectly capable of creating our own opportunities. At the same time, I am appalled at the way women are actively discouraged from feeling pleased with the size and shape of their bodies. You must be strong in the face of the unhealthy media messages we receive minute by minute. You must be strong and courageous in the face of advertising that is designed to make you feel weak, inadequate, and imperfect without the advertiser's product.

I will once again say quite firmly (with martini glass firmly in hand): If you are a size eight or a ten, relax and enjoy your life. Please don't think you need to become a six or a four. Achieve a healthy weight, and then stay there with your new indulgent eating habits. As much as I adore Chanel, I really don't have the classic Chanel body (which is a skinny, underdeveloped young girl, it would seem). I am never going to be a flat-chested and small-hipped woman. It just isn't going to happen. So I wear what I can—luscious black velvet pants, handmade spectator pumps, and a Chanel blazer instead of the classic suit design. Oh, and I have a lot of Chanel earrings, too, which fit perfectly, regardless of the size of my chest.

Earlier I was quick to point out what indulgence is not—it is not gluttony, not indolence; instead, it is recognizing your right to be happy and receive pleasure from food. Indulgence, I grandly stated in the first chapter is *the absence of fear when it comes to allowing yourself a pleasure, combined with the courage to declare that, henceforth, you will allow only the very best of everything into your life.*

You will allow only the very best of everything into your life. Isn't that a delightful vow to undertake? Not a vow of poverty, not a vow of chastity, but a vow of indulgence. Like buying the very best gin (oooh, and I think that would be Hendrick's), do allow yourself to buy the very best ingredients available, to become a habitué of farmers' markets and specialty food shops, to buy the very best chocolates, the very best and freshest organic heirloom tomatoes, handmade cheeses, free-range chickens, and baby spinach.

Remember, you are now a committed food snob. You do not eat food that is not up to your very high standards. Smile kindly at the gloppy chicken casserole your new neighbor offers up, but please take only a polite bite or two before turning away.

Can you see how this will begin to change every part of your life? Instead of a fat-bomb breakfast on the weekends, you will spend a lazy Saturday morning wandering the colorful aisles of the local farmers' market, deciding which of the freshly baked loaves of bread you should buy to toast with those newly laid eggs. Instead of an afternoon spent plopped on the couch, you'll spend it gliding effortlessly around freshly scraped ice at your local rink, moving in time to stirring violin music. Instead of a hurried meal pulled from the microwave and plopped on the table in front of the TV, you'll spend your evenings with good friends and good food, lingering late into the evening over a tiny glass of port and a hunk of dark chocolate.

Rediscover your own kitchen—cooking from scratch doesn't have to be difficult. I've included as many of my own favorite recipes as the publisher allowed in the last chapter of this book. You'll find that spending time in your own kitchen gives you a greater appreciation for what you are eating, and you have complete control over the portion size. With an empty martini glass at hand with which to measure out the right amounts, your restrained and refined approach will soon become second nature.

Once you've rediscovered your kitchen and the pleasures that lie within, please do begin to entertain more. Not only is the conversation more stimulating than when you are by yourself, you won't run the risk of leftovers calling your name from the refrigerator at two in the morning.

Living the Martini Lifestyle

 Feeling the need to go to a fancy restaurant? Ask yourself—what am I really hungry for? Am I hungry for a meal? Or maybe I just long for the chance to sit in a beautiful room where all is peaceful and calm. Why not drive past the restaurant and go to a museum instead?

Our hero at the table of moderation, Julia Child, recommends similar restraint when it comes to indulging. She suggests we look at it this way:

"An imaginary shelf labeled 'indulgences' is a good idea. It contains the best butter, jumbo-size eggs, heavy cream, marbled steaks, sausages and pâtés, hollandaise and butter sauces, French butter-cream fillings, gooey chocolate cake, and all those lovely items that demand disciplined rationing. Thus, with these items high up and almost out of reach, we are ever conscious that they are not everyday foods. They are for special occasions, and when that occasion comes we enjoy every mouthful."

Isn't that a lovely mental picture? That's a shelf I wouldn't mind being forgotten on for a week or two, just long enough to eat a bit of that gooey chocolate cake she has stashed there. And I would enjoy every mouthful, indeed.

Living the Martini Lifestyle

By now I hope that you are as fond of our food goddess, Julia Child, as I am. As a wonderful way to honor all she has done for food, for cooking, for eating, and for tall, strong women everywhere, why not make yourself a dinner of a lovely cut of red meat and some fresh vegetables, pour yourself a martini made from Gordon's gin, and read the Julia Child biography *Appetite for Life*, by Noel Riley Fitch. Red meat, gin, and Julia. What a marvelous way to pass an evening.

If you haven't been enjoying every mouthful in life, I believe that is about to change. You deserve to eat the food you want, rather than constantly denying yourself the best life has to offer. Instead of a body attained through vigilance (denying, counting, avoiding), wouldn't you rather have a body and a life attained through pleasure? Wouldn't you rather enjoy wonderful food, good conversation, delicious wines, and an active and elegant lifestyle that keeps you moving on horseback, on ice skates, or across the polished dance floor?

Living the Martini Lifestyle

Winston Churchill liked his martinis so very dry that his method involved pouring the gin in the glass, glancing briefly at the bottle of vermouth, and then getting back to business with his gin. Perhaps we too can adopt this Churchillian approach to foods—just glance briefly at the food and feel sated.

The Science of Self-Indulgence

Research shows that 95 percent of dieters who successfully keep off the weight exercise almost daily. Adopt one of my indulgent exercises and make it a part of your new life forever.

You've seen the many ways you can incorporate exercise into your life in a manner that will open you up to new experiences and new people, not leave you shut up and sweating alone inside a sterile gym.

I don't just want you to change your eating habits or the shape of your body; I want you to change the shape of your life. I want you to make a major change in what you think you deserve from life, to ask more of yourself and of the people around you. Surround yourself with people who not only support your weight goals and your new eating habits but who also support your image of yourself and what you can accomplish.

Slide off of life's barstool and create the life you dreamed of as a girl, with the clothes, the music, the flowers, the romance. You have the power to create all those things for yourself. No one will give you the body or the life you crave; you need to take responsibility and create it yourself.

Join with me now, take that racy new name, those lovely new clothes, and your new eating philosophy, and get out there into the big wide world and start drinking it in.

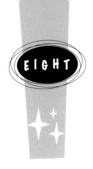

EIGHT

My Favorite Indulgences

It just doesn't seem right for me to encourage you to be a food snob and turn your nose up at most ordinary offerings and then not share the recipes for the very foods I enjoy most. Mind you, all of these recipes* fall into our rule of **Eat Only the Very Best** *and rely on fresh ingredients and modest kitchen skills. I hope you enjoy making these dishes and serving them with love to your friends and family, as well as yourself! Dining alone is a perfect time to pull out this cookbook and really do up something special. Why should you restrict your meals to a sad and solitary bowl of cereal when you are on your own? You absolutely deserve the best at every meal.*

---

*Okay, I confess: There is one cake recipe that uses a prepackaged ingredient or two, but it is so darn good that I didn't want to deprive you. When you bring it to a party just don't tell *anyone* what's really in it!

How much of this luscious food should you eat? Refined and restrained helpings, of course, fairly modest in size. The flavors, the colors, and the textures will help you feel satisfied quickly and able to stay in the modest-portion range with ease. If you eat the entire fresh fruit tart yourself, however, or pig out on Pashmina Pudding, don't come crying to me that you haven't lost weight, dearie. With each recipe, I am providing a standard serving size, but here is my advice: If a recipe says "Serves four," then on the Martini Diet, it should really serve six.

Now, pour yourself a tall, thin glass of something wonderful and enjoy!

SECTION I ~ A LITTLE SOMETHING TO START WITH: BEVERAGES, BREAKFASTS, APPETIZERS, SOUPS, AND SALADS

You can't just jump into a full dinner without a few things to serve beforehand, and I thought you might like a few extra ideas for sumptuous breakfasts. Who wakes up feeling creative in the kitchen? Not I. Instead, I rely on a small but carefully honed list of favorites with which to start my indulgent day. I love to entertain, so I've included my recipe for a fail-proof cocktail party, as well as a luscious drink recipe that will make holiday guests cheer your name.

recipes include

The Perfect Cocktail Party

Eggnog

Ice Cream Breakfast

Eggnog French Toast Soufflé

Sour Cream Waffles

Bourbon Cheese Straws

Hot Corn Relish

Savory Christmas Soup

Sweet Potato Vichyssoise

Suburban Chicken Stock

Century Farm Creamy Pea Soup

Granite Bay Cassoulet

Barbara's Roasted Carrot Soup

Creamed Spinach

Crispy Sweet Potato Wedges

I bunch red
seedless
grapes

I cup raw
unsalted
almonds

I pear,
left unpeeled,
cut into slices

I green apple,
left unpeeled,
cut
into slices

Cambozola
cheese (found
in the cheese
section near
the Brie)

Freshly made
baguette
toasts

The Perfect Cocktail Party

So much stress has been wasted on the idea of entertaining. It's very simple, really. Just stock the bar, polish your crystal, and put the following ingredients on a lovely platter next to some impressive paper napkins you pinched from your favorite bar. Bake the toast an hour before your guests arrive and your house will smell tantalizing. Instant party success, and no worrying.

[Toast]

To make the baguette toasts, buy one thin loaf of high-quality French sourdough and slice into ¼-inch (.63cm) rounds. Preheat oven to 350°F (180°C/Gas Mark 4). In a bowl, mix several tablespoons of high-quality olive oil with salt and pepper to taste, one finely chopped clove of garlic, and a handful of chopped fresh herbs, such as rosemary and sage. Using a pastry brush (or a sprig of rosemary if you are feeling rustic), slather this mixture onto both sides of the bread slices. Place on an ungreased cookie sheet and bake for 8 minutes, or until they begin to brown. Check often to make sure they do not burn. Remove from oven, and carefully flip over each piece and cook for another 5 minutes, or until nicely browned. Allow to cool on wire racks.

Serves four.

Eggnog

Real eggnog is extraordinary, unbelievably rich, and decadent. And it contains the calories of an entire meal, so plan your day accordingly. Serving real eggnog to your holiday guests will make them feel special, too. Anyone squeamish about raw eggs should be warned in advance, though. Although I am a bourbon drinker, when it comes to eggnog, there is a camp that is equally enamored of rum as an addition. Whichever most appeals to you, use it. And if you are serving children, do leave it out.

ingredients

3 cups (705ml) whole milk

1 vanilla bean

6 eggs

½ cup (115g) plus 2 tsp sugar

1 cup (235ml) bourbon (as desired)

1 cup (235ml) heavy cream

Freshly grated nutmeg

Pour the milk into a large pot and add the vanilla bean, split lengthwise so that the yummy seeds are exposed. Heat the milk and vanilla bean over medium heat until just below a boil. Remove from the stove, allow to cool, and then refrigerate, covered, until you are ready to make the eggnog.

Separate the whites from the yolks into two bowls. Cover egg whites and store in the refrigerator. Add ½ cup (115g) of the sugar to the yolks, beating slowly until it is pale and frothy. Slowly add bourbon while stirring. Whisk in the cream. Cover this mixture and refrigerate for 3 hours.

About 1 hour before you plan to serve the eggnog remove the egg whites from the fridge and allow them to slowly come to room temperature. Whip them until frothy, adding the remaining 2 teaspoons of sugar. Take the milk mixture out of the refrigerator and remove the vanilla bean. Mix the egg yolk mixture and the milk mixture, then gently add in the egg whites. Garnish with freshly grated nutmeg.

Serves four.

Cream of
Wheat (not the
quick-cooking
kind)

Whole milk,
as needed

Fresh peaches

French vanilla
ice cream

Pure maple syrup

Ice Cream Breakfast

Ice cream for breakfast? Certainly, when it is used as a topping for a bowl of Cream of Wheat. Years ago, I spent a long, cold winter in the woods of Sweden and fell in love with the creamy white porridge my cousin would make. I ate it topped with thick cream and lingonberry jam. Anxious as I was to head home to California after months of darkness, I was reluctant to leave without a big bag of this delightful cereal. Imagine my surprise when a sharp-eyed American friend identified my special treat—Cream of Wheat. Oh. Well, that certainly made it easier to buy on a regular basis.

Cook the Cream of Wheat according to the instructions on the box. Use milk instead of water. In the meantime, peel and slice the peaches. Ladle the cereal into bowls and top with peach slices, a modest serving of ice cream (this is breakfast, after all), and a drizzle of maple syrup. For an even more indulgent breakfast, instead of vanilla, use my favorite ice cream—Dulce de Leche from Häagen-Dazs. To die for.

Serving size varies, depending on the amount of Cream of Wheat desired (see box).

Eggnog French Toast Soufflé

I make this Christmas Eve and refrigerate it overnight, then pull it out and let it cook while my sons are opening their presents. It puffs up beautifully brown and makes an eggnogy custard around the bottom edges. Serve it with some richly browned sausages for a complete meal, and don't skimp on the real butter and maple syrup, please.

ingredients

I loaf
French bread, sliced

½ cup (115g)
butter, melted

4 eggs

¼ cup (55g) sugar

I cup (235ml)
heavy cream

I cup (235ml)
eggnog

I tsp cinnamon

I tsp vanilla

Butter a baking dish that will easily accommodate the loaf of bread and is pretty enough to be brought to the table as a serving dish. Place the French bread loaf into the dish and fan the slices slightly. Pour the melted butter over the bread.

Mix the eggs, sugar, cream, eggnog, cinnamon, and vanilla and pour it carefully over the bread. The point is to make sure the loaf is well soaked with the creamy liquid. I use a turkey baster to squirt the liquid over the bread a few times before wrapping it in plastic and refrigerating it overnight. The following morning I bring it out and let it warm up to room temperature (using the turkey baster a few more times to make sure the bread is thoroughly soaked).

Place it into a 350°F (180°C/Gas Mark 4) oven and bake, uncovered, for 45 minutes until it is beautifully browned. Serve with plenty of unsalted butter and pure maple syrup.

Serves four.

ingredients

1 ½ cups (150g) flour

1 tsp sugar

¼ tsp baking soda

½ tsp baking powder

½ tsp salt

3 eggs

2 cups sour cream

4 Tbsp butter, melted

Whipped cream

Fresh strawberries, blackberries, or blueberries to top

Sour Cream Waffles

You simply can't invite friends over for Sunday breakfast and have them go away hungry. These are a wonderful brunch offering and are perfect with lots of fresh berries and whipped cream. The recipe comes from my friend Rita Harris, who is a wonder in the kitchen.

Preheat the waffle maker. Mix together the flour, sugar, baking powder, baking soda, and salt. In a separate bowl, beat the eggs until they are a creamy lemony color, then blend in the sour cream. Stir the dry ingredients into the egg and cream mixture, and then add the melted butter. Mix well.

Bake according to the waffle iron's instructions. If adding fresh fruit, slap on a dollop of freshly whipped cream and decorate with a generous serving of berries.

Serves four.

Bourbon Cheese Straws

No, they don't actually have bourbon in them, but these cheese straws are a wonderful accompaniment to a big glass of small batch bourbon. It's a Southern thing, you see. Bourbon cheese straws are also a nice companion to a bowl of soup in the wintertime. Make these before a cocktail party and impress your guests with your devotion (to them, not to bourbon).

ingredients

1⅔ cups (190g) flour

1¼ tsp dry mustard

1 tsp salt

¼ tsp pepper

2½ cups (300g) grated Cheddar cheese

1 stick (115g) butter (room temperature)

2 Tbsp water, plus more as needed

Mix together the flour, mustard, salt, and pepper in a bowl. In a different bowl, mix the cheese and the butter until well blended. This can take some time, and will look a bit odd and lumpy. Don't be discouraged. Beat the flour into the cheese mixture, adding water as necessary to form a dough.

Turn the dough onto a floured kneading board. Knead it just a few times and then place a sheet of wax paper over the dough ball. With a rolling pin, roll the dough into a rectangular shape, about 12 x 9 inches (30 x 22.5 cm). Put the shaped dough onto a cookie sheet and refrigerate for 20 minutes.

Preheat the oven to 425°F (220°C/Gas Mark 7).
Remove the dough from the fridge and pull the waxed paper off before beginning to cut the straws. Cut the dough in half crosswise, and then cut it into smaller 6-inch-long strips. Transfer cut straws to a clean cookie sheet and cook for about 12 minutes. Check on them after 10 minutes to make sure they don't burn, as burned bourbon cheese straws are just no good. Let them cool on a wire rack.

Serves eight.

ingredients

1 Tbsp
olive oil

½ yellow onion,
peeled and
chopped coarsely

1 clove garlic,
peeled and
chopped coarsely

1 package
frozen corn
or four ears of
fresh corn

1 small tomato,
chopped

1 Tbsp butter

Hot Corn Relish

This is a very quick and flavorful side dish to serve with a thick juicy steak or a big drippy hamburger. I invented it so I'd have a substitute for the French fries everyone else in my family eats when we barbecue.

Pour the olive oil into a frying pan, add the onion and garlic, and begin sautéing over medium heat until onions begin to soften and brown. Add the corn, tomatoes, and butter. Continue cooking until the corn is also lightly browned, about 7 minutes. Serve warm on the side of grilled beef dishes.

Serves four.

Savory Christmas Soup

Tiresome as leftover turkey can be after a few days, what do you do with the leftover baked ham? I mixed this up out of sheer desperation a few years back but like it so much I sometimes intentionally bake a large ham in order to be able to make the soup. The best, most flavorful kind of ham is, of course, one of those sticky sweet brown sugar ones. Imagine how sumptuous a soup that will make.

Rinse the beans and put them in a pot filled with 8 cups (1880 ml) of water. Bring to a boil, turn off the heat, and let sit, covered for 1 hour. Drain and rinse a second time. Put the beans back into the soup pot and add fresh water, about 8 cups (1880ml). In a saucepan, cook the onion, bacon, and garlic until lightly browned. Add the onion, bacon, garlic, and bacon drippings to the beans and bring to a boil. Turn down heat and simmer for 2½ hours. Add the: curry powder, salt and pepper to taste, leftover ham, and Brussel sprouts. Cook another 30-45 minutes.

Serves six.

ingredients

1 bag small white beans

1 medium onion, peeled and chopped

5 strips bacon

4 cloves garlic, peeled and chopped

1 tsp curry powder

Salt and pepper to taste

As much leftover baked ham as you have, cut into bite-size pieces

Brussel sprouts or other leftover green vegetables

3 Tbsp butter

½ yellow onion, chopped

4 cups (940ml) chicken stock (see recipe on next page)

I cup (235ml) sweet white wine (like a Riesling)

2 large sweet potatoes, peeled and cut into chunks

Salt and pepper to taste

½ cup (120ml) whipping cream (optional)

Sweet Potato Vichyssoise

This is an incredibly creamy and flavorful soup that can be served either hot or cold. I love it cold as a weekend lunch, served with thick slices of fresh wheat bread slathered with butter. It is also a frequent first course for my Red Wine/Black Dresses dinner parties.

In a soup pot, melt the butter and sauté the onion for 10 minutes, or until brown. Add the soup stock, wine, and potatoes; bring to a boil. Simmer for 20 minutes or until the sweet potatoes are soft. Remove the soup pot from the stove and allow it to cool for 30 minutes (it makes it much easier to handle while processing). Using a food processor or blender, add the soup in small batches and purée until smooth. Once the entire batch is smooth and creamy, taste and adjust the seasonings with salt and pepper. You can add whipping cream (unwhipped) at this point to make it even richer, but I find that it is lovely without it.

Serves six.

Suburban Chicken Stock

Suburban chicken stock? Yes, because I believe that the most flavorful stock is made by using those rotisserie chickens that are now sold in suburban grocery stores everywhere. They are already so heavily salted and spiced that the broth it makes is heavenly. Buy one (two is even better) and serve your family roasted chicken for dinner, and then begin making your stock the minute dinner has ended. Your house will smell wonderful. I like to use it right away in a pot of soup or beans the very next day, but if this isn't possible it does freeze well for a month.

5 cups
(1175ml) water

1 to 2 leftover rotisserie chickens, including all bones and skin

Handful of carrots

2 cloves garlic, peeled and smashed

½ yellow onion, peeled and quartered

Any leftover vegetables from dinner

Combine all the ingredients in a soup pot. Bring to a boil and turn the heat down to let the stock simmer slowly for at least 1-2 hours. Remove from the heat and allow to cool for 15 minutes. Place a strainer over an empty soup pot and strain the broth, saving the remaining chicken and vegetables in the sieve. Set aside to cool. At this point I always put the stock in the fridge for use the following day (chicken fat and all). Once the bones and vegetables have cooled enough to be handled, I always pick through it and save any chicken meat for a dish of enchiladas or tacos. Discard the vegetables and bones.

Yields approximately 4 cups.

ingredients

2 cups (130g)
chicken stock

1 cup (235ml)
peas, fresh
or frozen

2 carrots, peeled
and chopped

1 potato, peeled
and chopped

1 yellow onion,
peeled and
chopped

2 cloves
garlic, peeled
and smashed

2 tsp curry
powder

1 cup (235ml)
heavy cream

Salt and pepper
to taste

Century Farm Creamy Pea Soup

Our family farm in Washington's Skagit Valley is a perfect spot to enjoy freshly picked peas. This soup is very easy and fast and can be made with either homemade chicken stock or canned broth and either fresh peas or frozen. Master this recipe and you will use it often.

In a soup pot, combine 1 cup (235ml) of the chicken stock with the peas, carrots, potato, onion, garlic, and curry powder. Bring to a boil and simmer until the potatoes are tender, about 15 minutes. Allow the soup to cool for 10-15 minutes before slowly adding to a food processor. Process in batches until the entire pot of soup is smooth. Add the second cup (235ml) of chicken broth and the cream and stir until smooth. Taste and adjust the seasonings with salt and pepper.

Serves six.

Granite Bay Cassoulet

Authentic French cassoulet takes several days to make and involves using every pot and pan in your kitchen. I adore it and seek it out in French restaurants and bistros around the world. When not traveling though, I wanted a way to enjoy a bowl without all the hassle of the traditional recipe. So this is my own invention, meant to be enjoyed on a winter's night in front of a raging fire with a glass of hearty red wine. One of these days I'll figure out how to make it even more authentic by adding duck. Until then, this does the trick nicely.

ingredients

1 package Great Northern white beans

4 cups (940 ml) chicken stock (see recipe for Suburban Chicken Stock, page 157)

1 large smoked sausage, chopped into 1-inch pieces

2 cups (220 g) leftover cooked chicken, shredded

1 cup (130 g) small carrots

2 Tbsp olive oil

1 onion, peeled and sliced

5 cloves garlic, peeled, smashed, and chopped

1½ cups bread crumbs

Rinse the beans and soak them overnight in a pot of water. Drain, rinse again, and discard the old water. Add fresh water to cover the beans, bring to a boil, and cook for 30-40 minutes until somewhat soft. Drain beans and return them to pot. Add the chicken broth. Add the sausage, shredded chicken, and carrots to the beans and stock. In a saucepan, heat the olive oil slightly and add the onion and garlic. Sauté until brown, and then add this mixture (including any leftover olive oil in the pan) to the bean pot. Gently stir all ingredients together; it should be quite soupy. Cook in a 350°F (180°C/Gas Mark 4) oven for 45-60 minutes. Remove from the oven and add a layer of bread crumbs to the top. Return to the oven and cook until crumb layer is browned and the beans are bubbly.

Serves six.

ingredients

5 pounds
(2275g) carrots,
coarsely chopped
(cut off the ends
but do not peel)

5 large onions,
peeled and
coarsely chopped

Olive oil as
needed

Chicken stock
to cover,
about 8 cups
(1880ml)

Fresh ginger,
to taste

Balsamic vinegar,
to taste

Herbs and spices
to taste, such
as dried
tarragon, thyme,
and pepper

1 cup crème
fraîche or
plain yogurt

Barbara's Roasted Carrot Soup

You've heard about Barbara Curtis, who runs the Slow Food Convivium in Lake Tahoe, California. An invitation to her kitchen is not to be missed, and some of my favorite food memories derive from that same cozy kitchen. When I asked her about a favorite recipe to share with the Martini Diet devotees, she offered up this scrumptious soup. And don't be afraid to really brown those carrots she says; the slightly charred skins give the soup its flavor. This recipe makes quite a bit of soup because, as Barbara says, "If you're going to work this hard, you might as well make a lot of it!"

Preheat the oven to 400° (200°C/Gas Mark 6). Place the chopped carrots and onions in a large oven-proof roasting pan and generously lace with the olive oil. Roast for 45-60 minutes, stirring and turning the vegetables every 15 minutes or so. You really need to char these a bit; let them get quite darkly browned.

Dump the roasted vegetables and extra olive oil into a large soup pot and cover with the chicken stock. Bring the soup mixture to a boil, then let it simmer slowly for 1 hour, until the carrots are very soft. Allow to cool slightly before processing, either with a wand blender (Barbara's method) or in batches with a food processor. Once the soup is creamy smooth, begin to season to your taste. Generously grate fresh ginger. Add vinegar 1 tablespoon at a time, tasting in between to decide how much of a bite you like. Add herbs and spices according to your own taste. Dried tarragon and thyme work nicely. Serve in bowls topped with a dollop of crème fraîche or plain yogurt.

Serves six.

Creamed Spinach

How can we eat thick and juicy steaks or roasts without this creamy food of the gods? Every steakhouse in America offers up a version (I'm fond of Morton's of Chicago myself), but I developed mine out of necessity to feed the Midwestern man I later married. Unable to find such an old-fashioned standard in the cookbooks I had available, I reached for an old collector's edition of the Fanny Farmer cookbook and figured out the basic idea. As my household is fond of Indian food, I like to add a bit of curry flavor to give it pizzazz.

ingredients

1 bunch
fresh spinach

2 Tbsp butter

1 Tbsp flour

Salt and pepper
to taste

½ tsp curry
powder or
garam masala

½ cup (120ml)
whipping cream
(regular milk can
also be used)

Add ½ cup water to a sauté pan, and cook the spinach quickly. Remove from the heat and drain. Leave in a strainer until needed. Melt the butter in the saucepan. In a small bowl mix together the flour and spices, and then add to the butter. Stir the spice mixture quickly and let it cook for 30 seconds or so before pouring in the cream and stirring into a smooth paste. Cook for a minute or so. If it seems too thick, add more milk or cream to achieve the consistency you like best. Add the cooked spinach and stir carefully, heating the spinach through. Serve immediately.

Serves four.

ingredients

4 large sweet
potatoes
(yams work
well, too)

2 Tbsp olive oil

Salt and
pepper
to taste

Crispy Sweet Potato Wedges

I'm fond of my root vegetables, have you noticed
that yet? (One big reason I don't do well on
carbohydrate-restricted diets.) These big crispy
wedges are wonderful next to thick slices of perfectly baked chicken. And what could be simpler?

Preheat the oven to 375°F (190°C/Gas Mark 5). Leave the skins on the
potatoes, but do cut the ends a bit. Slice the potatoes lengthwise into thin
wedges, about eight to a potato. Place the olive oil in a large mixing bowl
and sprinkle in the salt and pepper. I use a great deal of pepper in this
recipe when I make it. Mix well. Then add the potato slices and toss to
coat liberally. Place the wedges in a glass baking pan in one even layer.
Bake until cooked and slightly crisped, about 1 hour. Check for doneness
after 45 minutes and every 5 minutes thereafter.

Serves six.

SECTION II ~ MAIN DISHES

Now that you've had a cocktail and a little something first, perhaps a small bowl of creamy soup or a few red grapes and a bite of cheese and freshly baked toast, what's for dinner? Once or twice in my youth I flirted with vegetarianism (oh, who didn't I flirt with?), but as you will see from this list of meat-heavy recipes, it never really took. In fact, one day I plan to publish my dream cookbook, titled *Red Meat, Red Wine, Dark Chocolate*. I figure with those three I'll have enough variety in my diet.

recipes include

Global Village Fried Chicken

Quattro Fromaggio

Salmon in the Manner of Skagit Valley

Lemon Sage Roasted Chicken

Leg of Lamb

Roast Pork in the Manner of the Florentines

Lemon Spaghetti

Homemade Pizza

Dinner with Hemingway

Harvest Pork Roast

The Perfect Prime Rib Roast

Chicken and Corn Chowder with
Bourbon and Green Beans

Baked Chicken Breasts in Honey-Mustard
Marinade with Madras Curry

ingredients

2 chickens
(about 4 pounds
1820g each), cut
into pieces for
frying

2 cups (470ml)
buttermilk

2¼ cups
(260g) flour

1 Tbsp curry
powder

1 Tbsp cumin

Salt and pepper
to taste (I use
a lot with this
recipe)

Vegetable oil
or light olive oil
for frying

Global Village Fried Chicken

Once again, you will note the presence of Indian flavors in this Sander family recipe. Fried chicken just seemed so bland. Although I add spices liberally, the overall effect is pretty subtle in the finished product. After years of under-cooked fried chicken, I finally realized that baking it at the end is an absolute must. Nothing worse that being far away from home on a picnic and realizing the chicken you worked so hard on is way, way undercooked.

Put the uncooked chicken into a very large mixing bowl and pour the buttermilk on top. With your hands, move the chicken pieces around to make sure that they are well covered with the milk. Cover the bowl with plastic and allow the chicken to marinate in the refrigerator for at least 2 hours.

In an extra-large plastic freezer bag, pour in the flour and all the sea-sonings, seal, and shake from side to side to mix well. Pick the chicken out of the buttermilk, 2 or 3 pieces at a time, put them into the bag, seal, and shake until well coated. Remove and place on a plate, repeating until all the chicken is coated.

Preheat oven to 350°F (180°C/Gas Mark 4). In a large frying pan, heat the oil until ready (about 375°F/190°C), and carefully place the chicken in the pan. There should be enough oil in the pan so that it comes about halfway up the sides of the chicken. Fry both sides until golden brown, about 15 minutes each side. Watch carefully so that it does not burn. When browned, remove the chicken from the pan and drain on paper towels for a few minutes. Place in a large baking pan, spreading chicken out to just one layer, and bake for at least 30 minutes.

Serves eight.

Quattro Formaggio

Fellow writer and friend Lynne Rominger had a serious craving for this dish during a pregnancy and frequented a local restaurant weekly to get her fill. But one night she learned the restaurant was closing down for good! What would Lynne do? The owner kindly passed on the recipe so that Lynne could continue having a pleasant pregnancy. And Lynne herself has continued this act of kindness by serving it to our Red Wine/Black Dresses group.

ingredients

1 ½ cups each of the four cheeses—asiago, provolone, Parmesan, and Romano

1 ½ sticks (170g) unsalted butter

2 pints (950ml) heavy whipping cream

1 egg, beaten

Salt and pepper to taste

1 ½ pounds (685g) freshly cooked rigatoni

Grate the cheeses into a mixing bowl. Set aside. In a high-quality saucepan, melt the butter slowly. When the butter has melted, begin to add a bit of the cheese, a bit of the cream, whisking in between to keep it smooth, until all of the cheese and cream has been incorporated into the sauce. Continue cooking, but do not boil. You want the sauce to be thick and creamy. Add the beaten egg and whisk thoroughly; cook for just 1 minute more. Add salt and pepper to taste. When the sauce is ready, pour it over the hot rigatoni that has just been cooked and drained, and toss.

Serves six.

ingredients

1 large
salmon (skin on,
head and tail
removed)

2 large lemons,
cut into wedges

2 Tbsp soy sauce

4 Tbsp butter

Salt and pepper
to taste

Salmon in the Manner of Skagit Valley

This is the way my family has cooked their fresh-from-the-Puget-Sound salmon for generations. A lot of generations, eating a lot of salmon. Sometimes, a rogue will add an extra herb or two, or perhaps a splash of white wine, but the basic recipe stays the same. Serve with basmati rice and freshly picked corn for the best summer feast.

Make a sturdy pan out of several layers of heavy-duty foil, folding up the corners so that the sauce won't run out. Place the salmon in the middle and carefully squeeze the juice of the lemons over it. Pour the soy sauce over as well. Dot the salmon with butter. Salt and pepper to your heart's content. Place the foil directly on an outdoor grill. If you are cooking in an oven, put the foil onto a broiler pan, place on rack in the middle of the oven, and turn on the broiler. Monitor the salmon carefully, using a large spoon to continue to baste it with the sauce that develops. Cook at least 15 minutes, until just done in the middle, leaving it a tiny bit undercooked (salmon is cooked when it flakes).

Serves six.

Lemon Sage Roasted Chicken

Sage grows along my front walkway, and I am continually on the lookout for new ways to use it. This recipe was created in an effort to use up some sage, as well as some lemons that were getting tiresome. As to the best temperature for chicken, the debate rages on. Slow and low on one side, and high and fast on the other. For many years I did the 450°F (230°C) for 45 minutes thing, but I have lately gone back to the slow and low camp. This recipe is designed for the slow and low method; the herbs will burn under the heat.

Preheat the oven to 350°F (180°C/Gas Mark 4). Put the chicken in the center of the glass baking pan and pour the olive oil over. With your hands, rub the garlic and herbs all around the skin of the roast, pressing hard. Salt and pepper liberally. Cover the roast loosely with foil and bake for 30 minutes. After 30 minutes, remove the foil, and squeeze the juice of half a lemon over the chicken. Continue cooking for another 30 minutes. Baste liberally. After 1 hour, squeeze the second half of the lemon over the chicken and add the baby carrots to the roasting pan, stirring carefully to moisten them. Ten minutes before the chicken is scheduled to be removed (total cooking time after basting should equal 1½ hours), add the peas to the carrots and stir. Pierce the leg; when the juices run clear, the chicken is done.

Serves four.

ingredients

1 large roast chicken

2 Tbsp olive oil

4 cloves garlic, peeled, crushed, and chopped

2 tsp fresh rosemary, finely chopped

3 tsp fresh sage, roughly chopped

Salt and pepper to taste

1 lemon, cut in half

1 cup (130g) baby carrots

1 cup (130g) peas, fresh or frozen

10 cloves
garlic, peeled and
chopped

⅔ cup (155ml)
extra virgin
olive oil

1 cup (235ml)
zinfandel

Cracked
black pepper

Salt to taste

6-to 8-
pound leg of
lamb, visible fat
removed

Leg of Lamb

Of all of the wonderful smells that can emanate from a kitchen, the smell of a roasting lamb reigns supreme for me. Okay, so maybe it isn't so much the lamb as it is all that heavenly garlic. Served with tiny boiled red potatoes and butter, maybe the creamed spinach (see page 161)—ah, now that's a dinner!

Combine the garlic, oil, wine, pepper, and salt to make a marinade. Put the lamb into a large zip-lock freezer bag and pour the marinade over it. Close the bag and begin to turn so that the marinade covers it completely. Place the bag flat inside of a glass baking pan and refrigerate for 24 hours. Turn the bag every few hours to evenly marinate the meat. When you are ready to cook, remove the lamb and discard the marinade. Heat oven to 350°F(180°C/Gas Mark 4). Put the lamb on a rack in a large roasting pan. Sprinkle liberally with salt and pepper. Bake until medium rare, about 1½ hours. Let the roast sit for approximately 10 minutes before carving. I like my lamb on the rare side; hope you do, too.

Serves six.

Roast Pork in the Manner of the Florentines

Marlena de Blasi, writer and chef extraordinaire, has so many wonderful recipes in her book, *Regional Foods of Northern Italy,* that dazzle and delight that I wasn't sure just which of them to include here as my favorite. This roast pork, however, tops the list. It is a knockout dinner party dish, as your house will smell divine.

ingredients

1 7- to 8-pound (3185-3640g) loin of pork

½ cup (120ml) extra virgin olive oil

1 head of garlic, peeled and crushed

⅔ cup (33g) fresh rosemary

Sea salt and freshly cracked pepper

1 cup (235ml) white wine

Lemon wedges

Preheat the oven to 400°F (200°C/Gas Mark 6). Cut 1-inch (2.5-cm) incisions all over the pork. In a food processor, process the olive oil, garlic, and rosemary into a rough paste. Add generous amounts of salt and pepper. Massage the paste into the pork, refrigerate, and let it absorb the flavors for at least several hours. Place the pork in a pan and roast until the internal temperature is about 155-160°F (68°C–71°C). Baste the roast every 30 minutes or so to moisten. Total cooking time will equal 1½ hours, but it is most important to monitor the internal temperature of the roast. When done, let it sit for 15 minutes to rest. Rinse the roasting pan with the white wine and form a sauce with the juices. Serve the pork with a bit of sauce and a wedge of lemon.

Serves six.

ingredients

1 pound thin spaghetti noodles

½ cup (120ml) lemon juice

2 Tbsp lemon zest

¼ cup (60g) Romano cheese

2 Tbsp fresh basil, finely chopped

4 Tbsp butter

Salt and pepper to taste

Lemon Spaghetti

I've tried to get my children interested in this great dish by calling it "lemonade noodles," but the fact is, it is a fairly adult taste. This is very easy and fast to make and is terrific when served with grilled salmon or a plain roasted chicken.

Cook the noodles al dente, then drain. Pour them into a pretty serving dish and add the remaining ingredients, tossing well to melt the butter and distribute the other flavors. I like quite a bit of pepper with this. The black pepper and the lemon zest look very good together.

Serves six.

Homemade Pizza

Once you learn how simple and satisfying homemade pizza is, never again will you sit down to a commercial slice of pizza. Blech. You need three crucial things to make this recipe— a bread machine to mix the pizza dough, a wooden pizza pallet, and a pizza stone on which to bake it. I know, you have a lot of unused kitchen equipment and are loathe to add more. But I promise you, you will use them weekly once you've mastered this. Homemade pizza makes a very impressive appetizer for dinner parties, particularly if you put out bowls of ingredients and let your guests make up their own combos.

ingredients

crust

1 ⅓ cups (315ml) water

¼ cup (60ml) olive oil

½ tsp salt

1 tsp sugar

¾ cup (90g) flour

¼ cup (30g) cornmeal plus a handful

2 tsp yeast

[Crust]

To make the crust, dump the water, olive oil, salt, sugar, flour, ¼ cup cornmeal, and yeast into your bread machine and select the white bread setting. Let it go through the entire kneading and rising cycle once, and then turn it off and let the dough rise further. Give this part of the process 1 ½ hours or so. Don't let it knead the dough a second time.

Put the dough onto a well-floured board and knead it a few more times. Separate into three or four rounds, depending on how many pizzas you plan to make and how large you'd like them to be. Roll into a round crust with a roller and use your fingers to push into shape. Place the pizza stone in the oven and preheat to 400°F (200°C/Gas Mark 6). Scatter the handful of extra cornmeal onto the pizza pallet. This makes it easier to slide the pizza off the pallet and onto the stone. Carefully place the round crust on the pallet and begin to decorate with ingredients.

[Pizza]

Personally, I am not a fan of pizza sauce. Too gloppy, too tomatoey. Instead, just pour a tiny amount of olive oil into the center of the rolled-out dough and spread it lightly with your hands to the ends of the pizza crust. Then begin adding whatever ingredients you'd like.

For dedicated sauce fans, spoon a small bit into the center and spread it out in a thin layer with the back of the spoon. Layer on the cheese next before adding the meat and vegetable ingredients. Typical pizza ingredients, such as pepperoni, sausage, ham, and pineapple are raised to a whole new level when you've made your own dough.

Once you've decorated your pizza to your taste, place in the oven for at least 10 minutes. I like to check frequently after that, carefully lifting the edge of the pizza with a long spatula to test the crust for firmness.

[Topping choices]

I like to spread just a bit of olive oil, sprinkle with a few types of cheese, then add fresh tomatoes, garlic, and a liberal amount of pepper. Cook for 8 minutes, and then add a handful of fresh chopped basil and continue cooking until the pizza bottom is firm and browned. And lastly, "sit," as my dear friend Laura once advised. So I did. "No, not you! Get up and talk to your guests! The pizza, let the pizza sit for a moment or two before cutting it!"

The other incredible combo I enjoy most includes walnuts, bacon, brie, chopped apple, and black pepper. Spread on olive oil, sprinkle with a bit of the basic pizza cheese mixture (Parmesan and mozzarella), and then place big hunks of brie around the crust, partially-cooked bacon, and raw walnuts, then grind black pepper over all. Pull it out when cooked and toss a handful of chopped apples onto the top to finish.

Makes two medium pizzas; serves four.

Dinner with Hemingway

After the birth of our first son (around the time I posted that "wear more cashmere" note to myself), I realized that my life seemed so very unsophisticated, so terribly suburban. The food was so childlike—nursery food, the British call it. Lots of eggs and toast and mush. Sigh. But then one afternoon I was reading a Hemingway biography while Julian napped, and I realized how very often Hemingway himself seemed to be eating eggs. Of course, he was eating them in a bistro in Paris, and I clearly was not. But nevertheless, it suddenly gave more of a gloss to my eggy meals, and I decided that a fine meal of eggs and roasted potatoes had a great deal of panache, particularly when paired with a glass of good red wine.

ingredients

8 eggs

¼ cup (60ml) whipping cream

Salt and pepper to taste

1 Tbsp unsalted butter

1½ pounds (680g) Yukon Golds (any potato will do, really) thinly sliced

2 Tbsp olive oil

2 tsp fresh rosemary, finely chopped

4 cloves garlic, peeled and coarsely chopped

Handful cooked, chopped spinach (optional)

[Creamy scrambled eggs]

In a bowl, crack the eggs and add the whipped cream, salt and pepper. Melt the butter quickly in a heavy frying pan and add the egg mixture. Stir frequently over medium heat as they cook, until fluffy and just barely done. To give it a little color you can add a handful of cooked and chopped fresh spinach.

[Roasted potatoes]

Preheat the oven to 400°F (200°C/Gas Mark 6). In a bowl, combine the potatoes with the other ingredients and toss to coat thoroughly. Spread in one layer in a glass baking pan, and salt and pepper to taste. Bake for 30-45 minutes until the potatoes are nicely browned, checking frequently and stirring with a spatula to keep them crisp and coated with oil.

Serves four.

ingredients

1 boneless
pork loin
center-cut roast

2 cloves garlic,
peeled, crushed,
and chopped

1 onion, peeled
and sliced

1 large sweet
potato, left
unpeeled, cut
into thick slices

2 Tbsp olive oil

12 fresh Brussel
sprouts, ends
trimmed

2-3 Tbsp real
maple syrup

Harvest Pork Roast

When the weather begins to turn and the late autumn vegetables come in, what could be better than mixing up several with a homey roast pork? Add a bit of maple syrup and your family and friends will soon insist that this is their favorite comfort food dish. I like to add a few prunes, but have since reconsidered after reading Fran Leibowitz's wry comment that no one wants to happen upon an "unexpected series of prunes" in their food.

Preheat the oven to 325°F (170°C/Gas Mark 3). In a glass baking dish, place the roast, the garlic, the onion and the sweet potato. Drizzle with the olive oil and toss to coat. You may add a tiny bit of water during the baking process if the vegetables seem dried out. Keep the vegetables moist while they are browning. Cook for 1 hour, then add the Brussel sprouts. Stir to coat with the juices. Cook for another 15 minutes, then drizzle a healthy dose of maple syrup over the roast and the veggies. Stir the vegetables yet again. Continue cooking until the roast reaches 145°F (63°C) internally. Remove from the oven and allow to sit for 10 or 15 minutes.

Serves six (depending on size of your roast).

The Perfect Prime Rib Roast

My favorite meal is prime rib, creamed spinach, and garlic mashed potatoes. Real horseradish on the side, not the creamy stuff. A very large glass of cabernet. Mmmm, I can smell it all now. I'll give you the recipes for creamed spinach and garlic mashed potatoes in a minute, but first let's learn how to make an incredible prime rib every single time. Fact is, this meat is so expensive you do not want to screw it up.

Preheat the oven to 500°F (260°C/Gas Mark 9) or the highest setting that it goes to without broiling. Salt and pepper the fat of the prime rib. Place the rib bone side down in a roasting pan. Insert a meat thermometer (don't let it touch a bone). Place the roast in the hot oven and cook for 15 minutes. Reduce the heat to 350°F (180°C/Gas Mark 4) and cook for 15 minutes per pound. The meat should be at 125°F (52°C) for medium-rare. Let the roast rest for 15 minutes before carving.

Serves four to eight (depending on size of your roast).

ingredients

4 boneless, skinned chicken breasts

1 Tbsp butter

1 tsp salt

Black pepper to taste

1 white onion, chopped

3 cups (130g) yellow corn kernels (use fresh in the summer, but frozen is fine in winter)

¼ cup (60ml) bourbon

2 Tbsp flour

2 cups (470ml) chicken stock, heated

½ pound (225g) green beans, trimmed and cut into ½ inch pieces

1 cup (235ml) half-and-half

Chicken and Corn Chowder with Bourbon and Green Beans

Can you picture this? Soup, with hard liquor. This makes a wonderful meal in itself. What could be better on a cold winter night, served with Cheddar biscuits just out of the oven. Why not skip the dinner table entirely and sit wrapped in old quilts in front of a roaring fire, spooning it out of bowls and feeling so cozy. Why does it taste so good? Because bourbon is corn mash whisky. Too wonderful.

Rinse the chicken breasts and pat dry with paper towels. Cut into cubes. Melt the butter in a Dutch oven over high heat. Add the chicken, sprinkle with ½ tsp of the salt and pepper to taste, and sauté for about 4 minutes over medium heat. Try not to brown the chicken. Remove the chicken with a slotted spoon to a plate. Add the onion to the pan and sauté for about 3 minutes. Add the corn and stir for 30 seconds. Raise the heat to high and pour in the bourbon. Carefully ignite with a match and let the flame die out to burn off the alcohol. Sprinkle the flour over the onion and corn and stir for 1 minute. Add the hot stock and bring to a boil, stirring constantly. Add the green beans, the remaining salt, more pepper if desired. Return the chicken to the soup for 2 minutes and heat thoroughly to blend the flavors. Add the half-and-half, stir, and serve piping hot.

Serves six.

Baked Chicken Breasts in Honey-Mustard Marinade with Madras Curry

ingredients

½ cup (175g) honey

⅓ cup (80ml) Dijon mustard

2 Tbsp soy sauce

1½ to 2 Tbsp Madras curry powder

6 boneless chicken breasts, skin left on

Both my husband and I are mad for Indian food, so the smell of curry is a common thing in our kitchen. One of these days I'm going to learn how to make nan bread, that wonderful stuff they cook in tandoori ovens. I just don't see how I'm going to fit a tandoori oven in my kitchen, so until then we will use fresh pita bread to mop up the juices. And basmati rice is necessary, of course.

The day before, in a bowl, stir together the honey, mustard, soy sauce, and curry powder. Pour into a zip-lock plastic bag. Rinse the chicken breasts and pat them dry, then add to the marinade bag. Give it a good swirl to make sure the marinade has completely covered the chicken. Refrigerate until needed. When you are ready to cook, preheat the oven to 350°F (180C°/Gas Mark 4). Arrange the chicken breasts, skin side up, in an oblong baking dish pretty enough to bring to the table. Bake until cooked through, about 40 minutes. Serve from the baking dish, spooning sauce over each serving.

Serves six.

SECTION III ~ SWEET SOMETHINGS FOR ALL OCCASIONS

At last, we arrive at my favorite part. The berry tarts, the creamy puddings, the gooey cakes, the very things that make it necessary for me to indulge in a heavy exercise and activity regime in order to be able to zip up my well-worn jeans. I want you to indulge in the desserts (and the exercise) too, but do remember how very modest our portions are, how very restrained and refined we are in our approach to eating these goodies. If a pie usually serves eight, you'll need to share it with ten or even twelve friends from now on. Don't worry, they won't go away from your house hungry and disappointed. Instead, they'll thank you for keeping them in their small jeans, too.

recipes include

Sweet Olive Oil Cake

Caramel Toffee Swoons

Glazed Cardamom Biscuits

Chocolate Fudge Cake

Swedish Cream

Mexican Chocolate Bread Pudding

Lemon Pudding Cake

Coca Cola Cake

Boyfriend Cheesecake

Fresh Berry Tart

Betty Nan's Banana Bread

Pashmina Pudding

Sweet Olive Oil Cake

Fond as I am of the sticky sweet and gooey dessert, this mild and subtle cake is a pleasant respite from chocolates and caramels. The ingredients list might lead you to believe you are making a dish to serve with a savory meat, but in fact it all conspires to create a lovely summer dessert. Serve with fresh strawberries or sliced peaches and a spot of slightly sweetened whipped cream.

Preheat the oven to 375°F (190°C/Gas Mark 5). In a large bowl, beat the yolks with the sugar until they are pale in color. Fold in the rosemary and the zests and set aside. In another bowl beat together the ricotta, oil, and wine. Mix the flour and salt together and add to the egg/sugar mixture, alternating with the ricotta mixture in three doses, gently stirring in between. Beat the egg whites until stiff and fold into the batter. Pour into a 10-inch (25cm) buttered, parchment-lined springform pan and bake for 25 minutes. Then reduce the heat to 325°F (170°C/Gas Mark 3) and cook an additional 20 minutes. Cool the cake for 10 minutes on a wire rack before unmolding.

Serves six.

ingredients

5 eggs, separated

⅔ cup (150g) sugar

2 tsp rosemary leaves, very finely minced

Grated zest of one lemon

Grated zest of one orange

4 ounces (115g) fresh, whole milk ricotta

½ cup (120ml) extra virgin olive oil

¼ cup (60ml) late harvest, white wine (very sweet)

1½ cups flour

¾ tsp salt

ingredients

1 stick (115g) butter

⅓ cup (70g) brown sugar

1½ cups (150g) uncooked oatmeal (not instant)

2 eggs

1 cup (225g) white sugar

½ cup (60g) flour

1 tsp vanilla

One 14 ounce (400g) bag of wrapped caramels

½ cup (120ml) whipping cream

3 Heath bars (or any toffee bar), smashed into small pieces

Caramel Toffee Swoons

I developed this recipe in an effort to win the Quaker Oats "Best Oatmeal Cookie Recipe." I figured the name alone—Swoons—would get me the prize check. Alas, I seem not to have won the contest but am happy to encourage you to make these regardless. For an incredible treat, serve a freshly baked swoon with French vanilla ice cream.

Grease a 9 x 13 inch (22.5 x 32.5cm) glass baking dish; preheat the oven to 350°F (180°C/Gas Mark 4) .

In a small saucepan on the stove, over very low heat, melt the butter and brown sugar together, add the uncooked oatmeal and stir thoroughly. Set aside. In a bowl, beat the eggs and white sugar thoroughly. Blend in the oatmeal mixture, then add the flour and vanilla. Pour half of this mixture into the baking dish and bake for 15 minutes.

Meanwhile, unwrap the caramels and place in the top of a double boiler (please put water in the bottom part first), then add the whipping cream. Stir continuously until the caramels have melted nicely to form a thick sauce.

When the first layer has baked for 15 minutes, remove the pan from the oven and pour the caramel sauce over it. Add the rest of the oatmeal batter on top of it. It will look a bit like a cobbler at this point. Bake at 350°F (180°C/Gas Mark 4) for another 20 minutes. Remove from oven and spread broken toffee pieces over the top.

Swoons need to sit for at least 1 hour before you cut them.

Serves twenty-four (entire pan of brownies).

Glazed Cardamom Biscuits

This could have gone in the first section, as it is a delicious treat first thing in the morning. But the fact remains that I am not much of a morning bake. So these sweet biscuits get made more often in the afternoon and are best shared over coffee (save some of that dark roast!) with friends.

[Biscuits]

Preheat the oven to 400°F (200°C/Gas Mark 6). Blend together theflour, baking powder, salt, and baking soda in a mixing bowl. Add vegetable oil and stir. Add the buttermilk and stir. Turn the dough mixture onto a floured board and knead until smooth. Roll the dough into a rectangular shape, about 8 × 15 inches (37.5 × 20cm). Spread the butter generously across the dough. Mix together the sugar, cinnamon, and cardamom in a small bowl, and using a spoon, sprinkle it over the entire surface of the dough. Roll the dough lengthwise into one long and skinny roll, and cut into 2-inch slices with a butter knife. They should look like spirals from the side. Place them on their sides (spirals facing up) in a buttered baking pan. Bake for 15 to 20 minutes, or until puffy and brown.

[Icing]

While the biscuits are cooking, place the powdered sugar in a small bowl and slowly add the milk, stirring until you reach the desired consistency (it should be runny enough to pour, but not too thin). Let the biscuits cool for 10 minutes before pouring the glaze over them. Serve warm.

Serves four.

ingredients

biscuits

2 cups (230g) flour

1 Tbsp baking powder

1 tsp salt

$\frac{1}{4}$ tsp baking soda

$\frac{1}{4}$ cup (60ml) vegetable oil

$\frac{3}{4}$ cup (180ml) buttermilk

1 stick unsalted butter (needs to be soft enough to spread)

$\frac{3}{4}$ cup (170g) sugar

1$\frac{1}{2}$ tsp cinnamon

$\frac{1}{2}$ tsp freshly ground cardamom

icing

$\frac{1}{2}$ cup (60g) powdered sugar

3 Tbsp milk, or more as needed

ingredients

1 18.5-ounce (525g) package of devil's food cake mix

1 3.4-ounce (100g) package of instant chocolate pudding mix

4 large eggs

¼ cup (60ml) vegetable oil

½ cup (120ml) chocolate syrup (the kind you pour over ice cream)

1 cup (235ml) sour cream

1 cup (235ml) mayonnaise

½ cup (120ml) strong coffee

1 cup chopped walnuts or almonds (optional)

1 cup (175g) chocolate chips (optional)

Kahlua (optional)

Powdered sugar (optional)

Chocolate Fudge Cake

Can you keep a secret? I hope so, because I don't want you to bust me to the Slow Food folks on account of how this incredible recipe includes an ersatz ingredient or two. But it is soooo good I'm willing to look the other way, and I hope you are, too. My friend Rita Harris, who used to own a bakery called Chocoholics, shared this recipe with me not long ago. She in turn got it from her friend Betty, and we both hope you share it with your friends in the near future.

Preheat the oven to 350°F (180°C/Gas Mark 4). Spray a bundt pan with baking spray and dust it with the unsweetened cocoa. Combine all the ingredients except the chocolate chips and nuts. Add the chips and nuts, if using, after the batter is well blended. Pour the batter into the bundt pan and bake for 50 minutes or until the top of the cake is almost firm. Remove the pan from the oven and place on a damp kitchen towel to cool. Invert the cake onto a cake platter. Should you wish to frost this cake, just add a bit of Kahlua to some powdered sugar to make a thin glaze and drizzle it over the cooled cake.

Serves eight.

Swedish Cream

For some reason, I've always been shy about attempting recipes that used gelatin as an ingredient. I just always worry that I will do it wrong somehow. But Swedish Cream is worth the potential failure, I think. It is a pristine white dessert that is fantastic when paired with fresh berries that you've cooked for a few minutes in a saucepan with a bit of sugar and a splash of water.

Dissolve the gelatin in the water in a small bowl. In a saucepan, combine the cream, milk, salt, and sugar over low heat. When the sugar is dissolved, whisk in the gelatin mixture and heat until smooth and the gelatin is completely dissolved. Pour from the cooking pot into a large bowl (preferably using a pouring spout). Cool slightly, stirring occasionally, but do not allow the mixture to set. Add the vanilla and sour cream, stirring and folding. Pour the Swedish Cream into individual dessert dishes and chill, covered, for at least 6 hours.

Serves six.

ingredients

2 envelopes plain gelatin

¼ cup (60ml) cold water

2 cups (470ml) cream

1 cup (235ml) milk

¼ tsp salt

½ cup (115g) sugar

1 tsp vanilla

2 cups (470ml) sour cream

6 cups (300g) of sourdough bread, torn into small bite-size pieces

2 cups (470ml) half-and-half

3 pieces of Mexican chocolate

4-ounces (115g) bittersweet chocolate

½ cup (150g) raisins, plumped in hot water for 30 minutes

2 eggs

¼ cup (60g) sugar

Mexican Chocolate Bread Pudding

Hot Mexican chocolate is a wonderful thing on a cold winter day. Not just chocolate, it also has cinnamon and extra sugar added and is sold in grocery stores in a bright yellow package. You bust off a piece, shave the chocolate with a dull butter knife, and add it to milk warming on the stove. Heaven. And even more heavenly is a bread pudding made with Mexican chocolate. At Christmas I've used commercial eggnog instead of half-and-half for a seasonal twist. Serve with a vanilla dessert sauce.

Start the day before by allowing the bread pieces to dry out a bit. Spread them on a cookie sheet and air-dry, uncovered, for a day. When ready to begin cooking, warm the half-and-half in a saucepan until just below a boil, remove it from the heat and add both types of chocolate and the plumped raisins. Stir until the chocolate melts. In a separate large bowl, beat the eggs and sugar together, then add the chocolate mixture and stir thoroughly. Add the bread and stir until the bread is well soaked. Let the bread mixture sit for 30 minutes and stir again to make sure the bread is evenly soaked.

Pour into a buttered baking dish and cover with foil. Set that pan into a larger baking dish into which you can pour about 2 inches of boiling water (it should reach up the sides of the pudding dish but not to the top). Slide very carefully into a 350°F (180°C/Gas Mark 4) oven and bake for 15 minutes. Remove the foil and bake for another 20 minutes. This bread pudding is wonderful just out of the oven.

Serves six.

Lemon Pudding Cake

ingredients

¼ cup
(30g) flour

1 cup
(225g) sugar

½ tsp salt

2 eggs, separated

⅔ cup
(150g) milk

2 tsp grated
lemon zest

⅓ cup (75g)
fresh lemon juice

I can't always eat chocolate, caramel, or pie. Well, I probably could if I had to, but sometimes I crave the tart taste of citrus. My children are always pleased to see Lemon Pudding Cake headed their way. It is a nice, light dessert to finish off a summertime party, too. Serve with lightly sweetened whipped cream.

Set the oven rack in the lower third of the oven and preheat to 350°F (180°C/Gas Mark 4). Sift the flour, sugar, and salt into a bowl. In another bowl, beat the yolks lightly. Stir in the milk, lemon zest, and lemon juice, mixing until just blended. Beat the egg whites until stiff. Fold into the batter, which will be light and somewhat runny. Pour the batter into a 1-quart baking dish and set this dish inside another, larger baking dish. Fill the outer dish with 1 inch (2.5cm) of very hot water. Bake for 50-55 minutes or until the top is golden brown.

Serves six

ingredients

cake

2 cups (450g) white sugar

2 cups (230g) flour

½ cup (120g) vegetable oil

3 Tbsp cocoa

1 stick (115g) unsalted butter

1 cup (235ml) Coca Cola

½ cup (120ml) buttermilk

1 tsp baking soda

1 tsp vanilla

2 eggs

1½ cups (150g) miniature marshmallows

icing

1 pound (455g) powdered sugar

1 stick (115g) unsalted butter

2 Tbsp cocoa

⅓ cup (75g) Coca Cola

1 tsp vanilla

Coca Cola Cake

After I've spent so much time telling you the horrors of tacky food and snacking and soda, please overlook my hypocritical stance when it comes to Coca Cola Cake. I had it for the first time many years ago in a little Southern food restaurant in Franklin, Tennessee, and was so overwhelmed by the taste and texture that I had to hunt down the recipe.

[Cake]

Grease and flour a 9 x 13 inch (22.5 x 32.5cm) baking pan. Set oven rack in center of the oven and preheat to 350°F (180°C/Gas Mark 4). Combine the sugar and flour in a mixing bowl. In a saucepan, heat the oil, cocoa, butter, and Coke, stirring to dissolve the mixture; then bring to a boil. Remove from the heat and pour the hot mixture over the dry ingredients. Beat well.

Add the buttermilk, baking soda, vanilla, eggs, and marshmallows, and beat well again. The marshmallows will not dissolve, and the batter will be rather thin. Pour into the prepared pan and bake 30 to 35 minutes. Don't worry if the cake bakes unevenly. Frost while warm.

Serves six.

[Icing]

Place the powdered sugar in a bowl. In a saucepan, bring the butter, cocoa, and Coke to a boil. Pour the butter mixture over the sugar and beat in the vanilla. Spread immediately on the warm cake.

Boyfriend Cheesecake

How many times did I make this in high school? For every boyfriend, every month, and with red food coloring on Valentine's Day. Since then I have had countless cheesecakes that are fancier, that have more exotic ingredients, but hey, nothing comes close to a basic boyfriend cheesecake. Once you've tried it, you'll be making it for boyfriends every month too!

[Crust]

Combine the graham cracker crumbs, ½ cup (115g) of sugar, and butter and press into a pie pan.

[Filling]

Cream the cream cheese in a bowl until smooth, then blend in the eggs, ⅔ cup (150g) of sugar, and 1 tsp of vanilla. Stir until smooth, and pour into the prepared crust. Bake at 375°F (190°C/Gas Mark 5) for 20 minutes. Remove and let stand for 15 minutes. While it is cooling, mix the sour cream, the remaining 2 Tbsp of sugar, and the remaining 1 tsp of vanilla. Once the cake has cooled, pour and then spread this mixture on top and return to the oven. Raise the temperature to 425°F (200°C/Gas Mark 6), and bake for 10 more minutes.

Serves six.

ingredients

crust

2 cups (230g) graham cracker crumbs

½ cup (115g) sugar

1 stick (115g) butter

filling

2 8-ounce (450g) packages cream cheese

2 eggs

⅔ cup (150g) plus 2 Tbsp sugar

2 tsp vanilla

1 cup (235ml) sour cream

ingredients ✳

crust

1 cup (115g)
flour

½ tsp salt

Grated zest of
1 lemon

1 Tbsp sugar

5 Tbsp unsalted
butter, cut into
small pieces

3 Tbsp milk
or cream

1 egg yolk,
beaten

filling

4 cups
(480-800g)
fresh seasonal
fruit such as
strawberries,
raspberries,
blackberries,
peaches, or
nectarines. (I
like to combine
a berry of some
sort with a few
peaches or
nectarines.)

2 Tbsp freshly
squeezed
lemon juice

2 Tbsp flour

½ cup (115g) plus
1 Tbsp sugar

Fresh Berry Tart

Despite my deep and abiding love of pie, I'm not much of a pie baker. Crisps and cobblers, no problem, but a pie has that tricky crust thing going. I learned to make this simple tart crust a few summers ago and since then have filled it with all manner of fruits. It is amazing, and now I wonder just what scared me about pastry for so long. Serve with the richest, creamiest vanilla ice cream you can find.

[Crust]

Combine flour, salt, zest, and sugar in a mixing bowl. Cut in the butter until the mixture is crumbly. Stir in the milk and egg yolk and form the dough into a ball. On a floured board, roll the ball into a disk, cover with plastic wrap, and put in the refrigerator for at least 30 minutes.

[Filling]

Combine the fruit, lemon juice, 1 Tbsp of flour, and ½ cup (115g) of sugar. Stir well. When the dough is firm enough, put on a floured board and roll into a nice round shape, about 10 inches (25cm) in diameter. Place on a buttered baking sheet with an edge in case it bubbles (which it always does). Spoon the fruit filling onto the center of the tart, mounding nicely. Fold the sides of the dough circle inward, forming a nice tucked envelope edge to hold the fruit in as it bakes. Dust around the pastry edges with the remaining 1 tbsp of sugar. Bake at 375°F (190°C/Gas Mark 5) for about 30 minutes, or until the crust is browned and the fruit is bubbling. Let it cool a bit before serving.

Serves four.